Manual of Skin Surgery

MANUAL OF SKIN SURGERY

A Practical Guide to Dermatologic Procedures

David J. Leffell, M.D.
Associate Professor of Dermatology, Plastic Surgery
and Otolaryngology
Yale University School of Medicine
New Haven, Connecticut

and

Marc D. Brown, M.D.
Associate Professor of Dermatology
University of Rochester Medical Center
Rochester, New York

WILEY-LISS
A JOHN WILEY & SONS, PUBLICATION INC.
New York • Chichester • Weinheim • Brisbane • Singapore • Toronto

The text is printed on acid-free paper.

Copyright © 1997 by Wiley-Liss, Inc.

Published simultaneously in Canada.

All rights reserved. This book is protected by copyright. No part of it, except brief excerpts for review, may be reproduced, stored in a retrieval system, or transmitted in any form or by any means, electronic, mechanical, photocopying, recording, or otherwise, without permission from the publisher. Requests for permission or further information should be addressed to the Permissions Department, John Wiley & Sons, Inc., 605 Third Avenue, New York, NY 10158-0012.

While the authors, editors, and publisher believe that drug selection and dosage and the specification and usage of equipment and devices, as set forth in this book, are in accord with current recommendations and practice at the time of publication, they accept no legal responsibility for any errors or omissions, and make no warranty, express or implied, with respect to material contained herein. In view of ongoing research, equipment modifications, changes in governmental regulations and the constant flow of information relating to drug therapy, drug reactions, and the use of equipment and devices, the reader is urged to review and evaluate the information provided in the package insert or instructions for each drug, piece of equipment, or device for, among other things, any changes in the instructions or indication of dosage or usage and for added warnings and precautions.

Library of Congress Cataloging-in-Publication Data

Leffell, David J.
    Manual of skin surgery : a practical guide to dermatologic procedures / by David J. Leffell and Marc D. Brown.
      p.   cm.
    Includes bibliographical references.
    ISBN 0-471-13411-2 (paper : alk. paper)
    1. Skin—Surgery. I. Brown, Marc D. II. Title.
    [DNLM: 1. Skin Diseases—surgery. 2. Skin Diseases—diagnosis.
  3. Skin—surgery. 4. Ambulatory Surgery—methods. 5. Dermatology—methods.
  WR 140 L493m 1997]
  RD520.L43   1997
  617.4'77—dc20
  DNLM/DLC
  for Library of Congress   96-30884
                                                                           CIP

Printed in the United States of America

10 9 8 7 6 5 4 3 2 1

To our wives, Cindy and Susan
To our children,
Alexander and Dahlia,
and
Marian and David

Contents

Preface ix

1 Introduction 3

2 Diagnosis 7
Defining the Lesion 7
Studying the Lesion 16
Common Skin Lesions 17
    Skin Cancers and Precancerous
      Lesions 17
    Common Benign Lesions 26

3 Practical Anatomy 31
Relaxed Skin Tension Lines 32
Regional Considerations 34
    Mouth 34
    Nose 34
    Ears 35
    Eyes 36
    Scalp 37
    Neck 37
    Back and Chest 37
    Upper Extremities 39
    Lower Extremities 40
    Superficial Anatomy 40

4 Wound Healing 51
Phases 51

5 Skin Biopsy 61
Incisional versus Excisional
  Biopsy 62
Shave Biopsy 63
Curette Biopsy 68
Scissors Biopsy 70
Punch Biopsy 70
Excisional Biopsy Technique 71
Special Considerations 75
Biopsy Record Keeping 80

6 Local Anesthesia 83
Chemistry and Classification 83
Local Additives 85
Allergic Reactions 86
Adverse Effects and Drug
  Interactions 87
Local Anesthesia Technique 88
Topical Anesthesia 93
Tumescent Anesthesia 94
Preanesthesia Medications 95

7 Surgical Instruments 99
Scalpels 100
Needle Holders 103
Forceps 105
Skin Hooks 105
Hemostats 107
Scissors 108

Curette 111
Miscellaneous Instruments 113
Instrument Care 113
The Surgical Suite 115

8 Wound Closure Materials 121
Absorbable Sutures 123
Nonabsorbable Sutures 126
Needles 128
Staples 131

9 Patient Preparation 133
Indications 133
Medical History 134
Patient Evaluation 138
Prophylaxis 141
Pacemakers 143
Blood Thinners 143
Dressings 146

10 Basic Excisional Surgery 149
Planning the Excision 149
Marking the Lesion 151
The Ellipse 152
Anesthesia 153
Drape and Preparation 154
Procedure 156
Wound Closure 162
Lazy S Repair 171

11 Surgical Complications 181
Bleeding 181
Infection 189
Necrosis 194
Dehiscence 196
Other Postoperative Problems 198

12 Special Topics in Dermatologic Surgery 205
Melanoma 205
Lentigo Maligna 209
Nevi 210
Skin Cancer 213
Mohs' Surgery 212
Cysts 217
Keloids and Scars 219
Lipomas 219
When to Refer 221

13 Risk Management 223
Informed Consent 224
Documentation 226
Confidentiality 228

Appendix I Action Guides 229
Skin Biopsy 230
Pigmented Lesions 231
Basal Cell Cancer 232
Squamous Cell Cancer 233
Complications 234

Appendix II Vendors for Dermatologic Surgery Suite 235

Further Reading 239

Index 241

Preface

At a time when the medical marketplace is inundated with textbooks on all aspects of health care, one might ask how a new volume on a well-known subject can be justified. In surveying the literature in dermatology, it is clear that the expanding field of dermatologic surgery is probably not comprehensively served at the introductory level. Specifically, there is no single volume which, in a brief and graphically engaging fashion, provides essential information necessary to develop skills in basic skin surgery.

Skin surgery, in its broadest sense, is a discipline that transcends specialties. Primary-care physicians including general practice physicians, internists, pediatricians and dermatologists, ear, nose, and throat surgeons, plastic surgeons, general surgeons, and others, all perform skin surgery. The skin is the most accessible organ and therefore the one that is most readily operated upon when needed.

The purpose of this book is to consolidate in one location the best practical teaching that is available regarding excisional cutaneous surgery. It is written from the vantage point of the authors who are schooled in dermatology. Our perspective on surgery of the skin is necessarily different from that of individuals raised in the surgical specialties. However, cutaneous surgery represents a substantial component of any dermatologist's practice, and dermatology has been a growing surgical specialty for many years. It is in this context that dermatologists have combined their special knowledge of the biology and pathology of the skin, and their surgical skills to allow for conservative, reasoned, and efficient surgical procedures.

Because dermatology is primarily an office-based specialty, we are able to present to you information in this text that will allow you to become an efficient office skin surgeon. In this era of constrained medical resources, when every government agency is clamoring for more efficient office-based care, we believe that this book can serve as your passport to that world of medicine that is increasingly in demand. We have attempted to make the information in this book lively, easy to read, and easy to reference in an ongoing fashion. Much of the scientific basis of the knowledge presented here is available elsewhere. This book is intended to be a very practical "how-to" manual and presumes the reader is knowledgeable in the substantiating science.

In many ways, this book represents the culmination of one aspect of our professional development. We would like, therefore, to thank one individual who played a very special role in that process. Neil A. Swanson, M.D., chairman of dermatology at the University of Oregon, trained both of us in surgical dermatology in the late 1980s. He is not only a superb teacher and devoted mentor, but an individual with whom we have developed a long, close, and rewarding relationship. Were we not married with families, we would have dedicated this book to him. We urge you to review his *Atlas of Cutaneous Surgery* as it was the first to present a systematic method for learning procedures described in this book. In addition, the texts by Bennett and by Salasche are landmarks in defining the specialty of cutaneous surgery. The authors have graciously given permission for us to use many of their figures in this book and for this we thank them.

This volume represents the information we have developed and passed on to medical students, residents and other physicians who have been interested in learning approaches to skin surgery. The elliptical excision is the workhorse of skin surgery and is the central focus and raison d'etre of this text. Some basic diagnostic information is provided and anatomy is briefly reviewed in a very pragmatic fashion. Patient preparation, surgical suite set-up, wound care and complications are all addressed in the context of the fusiform excision. The principles that underly this ubiquitous procedure are applicable both to advanced procedures like flaps and grafts and to simpler procedures like skin biopsy.

We hope that you will find the information in this text helpful and that it will allow you to progress with skin surgery to a rewarding degree. Please communicate with us any suggestions regarding improvements or changes.

New Haven, Connecticut DAVID J. LEFFELL, M.D.
Rochester, New York MARC D. BROWN, M.D.

Acknowledgments

In our chapters we repeatedly emphasize the importance of attending to all the patient's needs. Although some would consider skin surgery relatively minor, the degree of anxiety that patients have highlights the importance of listening to the patient and addressing all concerns. No individuals have been better teachers in this regard, nor better colleagues than the nurses and staff with whom we have had the good fortune to work at Yale. Diana Glassman, R.N., Anne McKeown, R.N. and Kristina Kline, R.N. are superior professionals who have taught much about caring for patients. Jackie Antunes, Pat Napoletano, and Lezlie Roark demonstrate through their commitment to our patients that it is indeed the team approach that benefits patients most. At Rochester, Georgette Ferris, R.N. complements her colleagues at Yale with her commitment and professionalism.

This book was written for the student, resident and physician who would like to explore excisional skin surgery. It is to our residents and students that we owe a special debt of appreciation. Through ongoing inquiry and curiosity, and a refusal to accept our teaching as dogma, our residents keep us honest and force us always to question our assumptions. Review of the manuscript has been an especially important aspect of ensuring that the text and features accomplish our goal. Several colleagues have taken the time to review the manuscript and offer many useful suggestions. Linda Zimmering, M.D., a family practice doctor in Toronto and John Oppenheimer, M.D., an internist in Sag Harbor New York gave a primary care physician's perspective. Jean Bolognia, M.D. a colleague and teacher at Yale whose breadth of knowledge in dermatology is enormous, offered highly valuable advice. Others from Yale who are now colleagues, including Irwin Braverman, M.D. and Aaron Lerner, M.D., taught me (DJL) dermatology with enthusiasm and wisdom and for this I am grateful. We continue to learn from our many

Acknowledgments

colleagues in plastic surgery and from Clarence Sasaki, MD, Chief of the Section of Otolaryngology at Yale. Our personal appreciation is also due the many dermatologists, surgeons, and primary care physicians of Connecticut, upstate New York, and the surrounding regions, who through their kind referral of patients, have made it possible for us to care for them, and teach additional generations of physicians.

Also, we thank George Blackburn and Joy Deloge of Yale and Mary Lou Williams of Rochester for expert secretarial assistance and commitment to this project.

Manual of
Skin Surgery

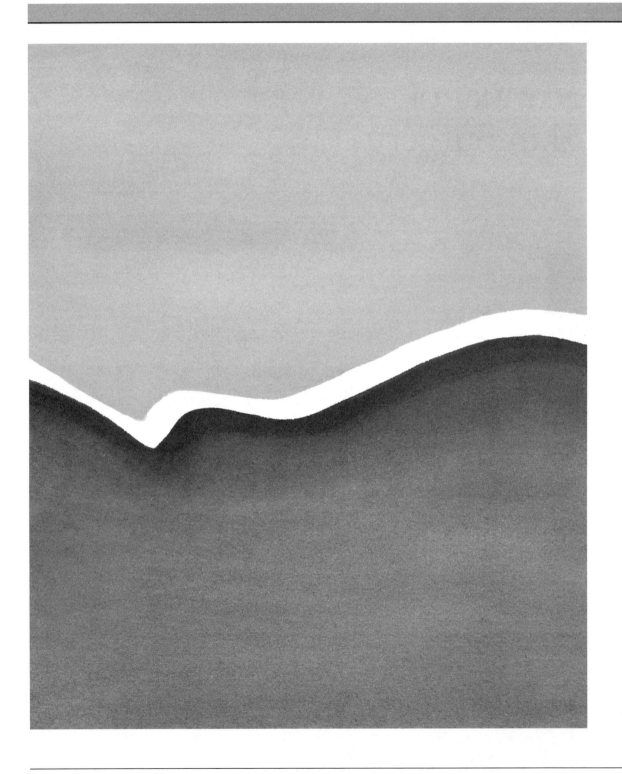

1

Introduction

As the population ages the incidence of dermatologic disease requiring surgical intervention increases. For example, the incidence of malignant melanoma, a cancer easily treated in the office in its early stages, rose from 4.5 per 100,000 in 1970 to 13.2 per 100,000 in 1991. Although the disease affects younger people to an increasing degree, malignant melanoma is still a cancer of older patients. It is estimated that in 1997 there will be approximately 34,000 new cases of melanoma and over 7,000 deaths from the disease. The management of melanoma, nonmelanoma skin malignancies such as basal cell and squamous cell cancer, and benign tumors of the skin will continue to fall to the dermatologist and other office-based physicians who can provide surgical services in the most cost-effective fashion. For these reasons, there is an almost unquenchable thirst for information on how to perform office skin surgery safely, effectively, creatively, and most importantly, competently.

This volume has two modest goals: first, to teach the elements of excisional skin surgery in a practical fashion to the medical student, resident, and practicing physician; and second, to convey subtleties of the field of cutaneous surgery that are already known to serious practitioners of the art. To achieve this end, the book has been structured in a relatively traditional fashion but includes technical sidebars known as "pearls." These pearls are really helpful tips and tricks of the trade that have become part of the oral tradition of dermatologic surgeons. We hope you will find it possible to pick up this book even for a moment and come away with information about excisional surgery that will enhance the care of your patients.

Introduction

Initial chapters on diagnosis, pertinent anatomy (which is always hard to make exciting), and wound healing give way, in logical sequence, to chapters including perioperative preparation and assessment, operative technique, and postoperative care.

While this book is primarily about technique and is intended to allow you to get up to speed quickly, dermatology has always been more global than just a therapeutic or diagnostic specialty. What distinguishes dermatologic surgery from its close cousins such as plastic surgery is the special emphasis placed on diagnosis and an understanding that the procedure performed on the patient depends on the clinical diagnosis. For this reason, a richly illustrated chapter on diagnosis is included. It concentrates on those conditions amenable to surgical intervention.

In this day and age of specialization, as a host of procedures now reflect back on the office-based physician, it is time to consolidate those aspects of technique and care that specialists have perfected for the benefit of the patient through their commitment, skills of observation, and creativity. A section on special topics in dermatologic surgery includes a practical guide to the management and work-up of melanoma, the indications for Mohs' surgery, and the approaches to common dermatologic ailments that have surgical solutions. In the appendix, clinical pathways are provided as flow diagrams to help you approach each clinical situation in a comprehensive and efficient fashion.

We hope that this manual will serve as a repository of information that is truly new to the reader and of great practical help. In the end, this book aims to improve the care you provide to your patients. As more and more is required of all physicians, we must become more demanding about our sources of information. This manual seeks to provide all that is good in dermatologic surgery, but it is important to attend courses on continuing medical education and, ideally, to study in the office or surgery suite along with experienced dermatologic surgeons. Our field is a peripatetic one: we borrow techniques, knowledge, and our understanding of the biological processes from all quarters of the expansive field of medicine. Each time we incise a patient we rely on new information developed by basic scientists, clinical researchers, and biomedical engineers. Importantly, surgery of the skin is the domain of no one specialty. It is the province of the skilled practitioner whether a dermatologist, family physician, plastic surgeon, or general surgeon.

As you proceed to develop skill and judgment in excisional dermatologic surgery, it is essential to remember always that the patient comes first. Whatever the distractions of modern daily practice, whatever the disappointments and frustrations of practice administration, whatever the stresses of fear of litigation, and whatever the concerns about the future of your professional life, you will be an excellent surgeon if you are first a superb doctor.

There is no doubt that skill can vary substantially from physician to physician. Surgical success in particular is dependent on a range of factors including hand/eye coordination, dexterity, ability to handle tissue, and most importantly and beyond our control, the native healing tendencies of the patient. The most critical factors for successful practice in office surgery, as in every other aspect of medicine, are judgment and availability. Beyond that, compassion, empathy, and the ability to put yourself in the patient's position while he or she is in your office is what will distinguish the reader of this book from his or her colleagues.

Our goal has been to help you build a solid foundation in the pursuit of clinical excellence in an exciting and fulfilling branch of dermatology. We hope we have done that challenge justice.

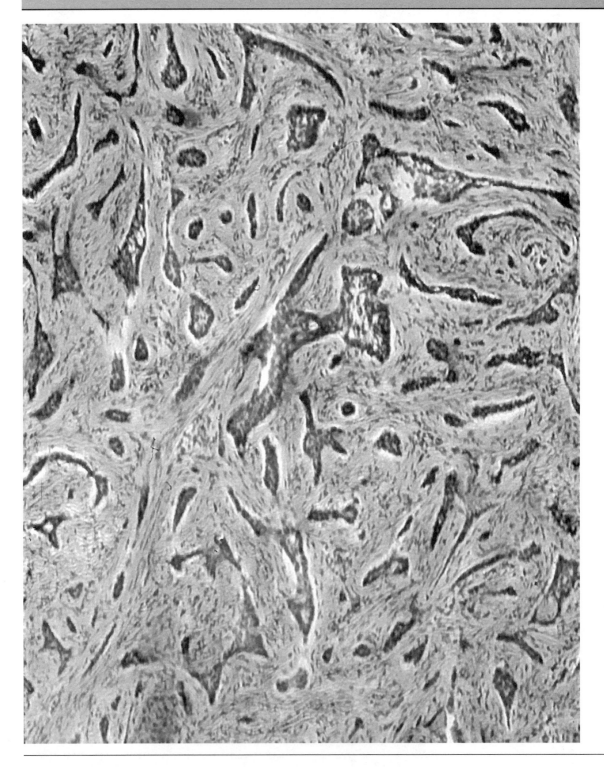

2

Diagnosis

The skills of skin surgery are geared to two specific goals: first, the diagnosis of specific skin lesions, and second, the treatment of those particular skin lesions. In order to develop optimal surgical skills it is important to have a thorough understanding of the terminology, microscopic and clinical presentation, and behavior of the skin lesions you are likely to see in practice.

Historically, dermatology was a field that relied heavily on the descriptive strength of Latin. Often it was alleged that the complexity of the language was merely a veil that concealed our lack of understanding of the diseases so described. In fact, the science of dermatology has progressed substantially in the past 20 to 30 years, but the language of dermatology remains firmly planted in its Latin roots. It is critical in our conversations with colleagues that we are certain we are all speaking the same language. In this chapter we review terminology and provide clinical examples of the common lesions that you are likely to encounter. Often the biopsy technique you select will depend on your appraisal of the lesion under consideration.

DEFINING THE LESION

All skin lesions have specific correlates with microscopic depth. An image of the miroscopic cutaway of the skin is important to keep in mind as the terminology used to describe lesions is approached

Diagnosis

[Figure 2-1]. For descriptive purposes, lesions are either confined to the epidermis, extend into the dermis, or involve the subcutis (deep dermis and fat). Herewith are the basic descriptive terms used in dermatology accompanied by clinical examples.

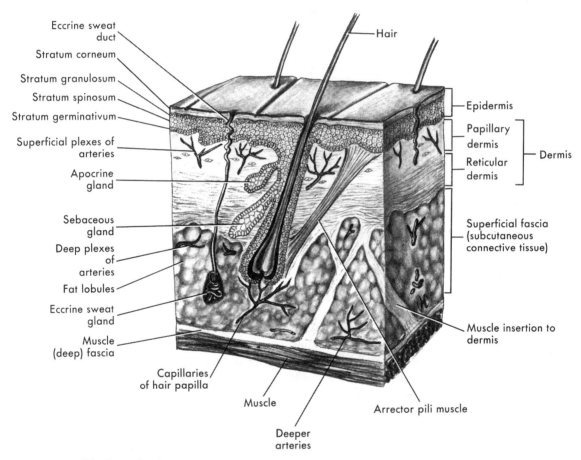

Figure 2-1. Skin Cross Section
The skin represents a complex multilayer structure organized to permit rapid and effective healing upon injury. The epidermis consists of a layer of basal cells that give rise sequentially to more squamous-appearing cells. The horny layer of the epidermis represents dead keratinized cells and keratin, a protein product of squamous cells. The vascular supply of the skin terminates in fine capillaries that perforate the papillary dermis and supply the complete organ. Reprinted with permission from Bennett, Richard G., 1988, Fundamentals of Cutaneous Surgery, *Mosby, St. Louis, MO. p. 19.*

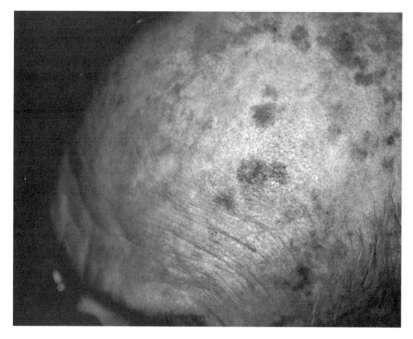

Figure 2-2. Solar Lentigo
Some of the solar lentigos on the forehead of this elderly man represent macules. They are variegated in color and flush with the surrounding skin. Macules are generally smaller than 1 centimeter. These are distinct from patches which are larger than 1 centimeter and are flat.

MACULE. A small flat patch of skin that varies from the surroundings by a difference in color or surface texture and is usually less than 1 cm in largest diameter. An example is an age spot or a sun spot [Figure 2-2].

Brown macules. Actinic lentigo (freckle), lentigo maligna, Becker's nevus, cafe au lait spot, lentigo, pigmented nevi.

Brown macules on palms and soles. Acral lentiginous melanoma, junctional nevus, talon noir [Figure 2-3].

Hypopigmented macules. Vitiligo, halo nevus [Figure 2-4], post-inflammatory hypopigmentation. This latter entity is important to recognize as it may develop following various surgical interventions.

Blue macules. Mongolian spot, nevus of Ota [Figure 2-5] or Ito—these are congenital. Acquired conditions: blue nevus, malignant melanoma, tattoo.

Red macules. Usually represent exanthems and are not pursued surgically except for biopsy or if they represent precancerous lesions.

Diagnosis

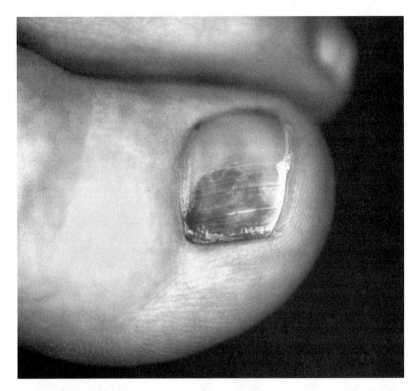

Figure 2-3. Talon Noir
Black nail must raise the suspicion of melanoma. The majority of talon noir are secondary to trauma and represent the by-products of the degradation of extravasated blood.

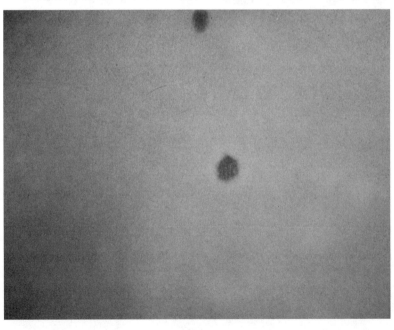

Figure 2-4. Halo Nevus
This benign nevus is characterized by central pigmentation surrounded by an area of depigmentation. It may be considered a variegated pigmented macule. Its significance lies in the fact that the area of depigmentation most likely represents an inflammatory reaction by the body in an attempt to destroy nevus cells that may be transforming. Note the superior normal-appearing nevus lacks the halo.

Defining the Lesion

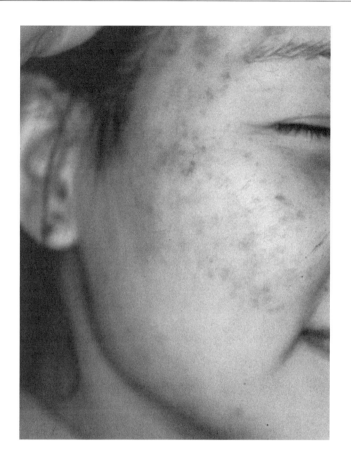

*Figure 2-5. Nevus of Ota
Diffuse pigmentation is represented and is best described as a patch of pigmentation. The color is slate gray.*

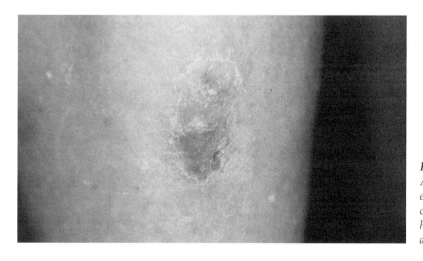

*Figure 2-6. Plaque
A plaque is a raised patch. This example of superficial basal cell carcinoma demonstrates a hyperkeratotic surface against an erythematous background.*

Diagnosis

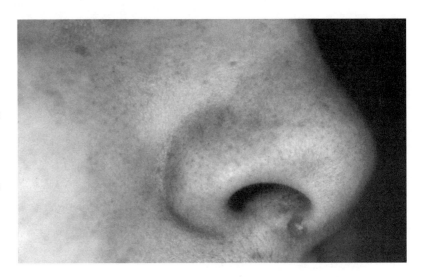

Figure 2-7. Papule
A papule is a well-defined lesion raised above the surface of the skin that is usually dome shaped. It is less than 1 centimeter in diameter. A nodule is a papule that is 1 centimeter or greater. In this case, the clinical presentation is that of a nevus, a benign mole that consists of nevus cells extending from the dermis and rising above the surface of the skin.

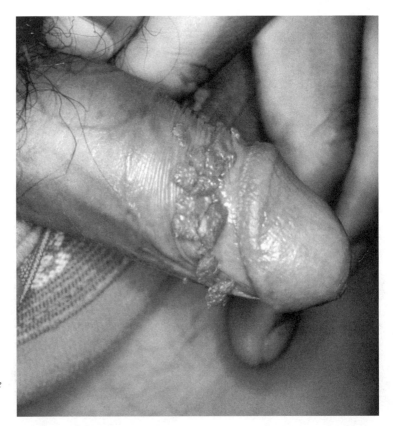

Figure 2-8. Condyloma
Condyloma appear as multiple papules that are flesh colored and in some cases pedunculated. Condyloma are amenable to a variety of therapies. Warts in general have a wide range of clinical presentation.

PATCH. A macule greater than 1 cm.

PLAQUE. A raised version of a patch [Figure 2-6].

PAPULE. An elevated bump on the surface of the skin, usually considered to be less than 1 cm.

Flesh-colored papules. Nevi [Figure 2-7] skin tags, condyloma [Figure 2-8], comedone, molluscum contangiosum, basal cell cancer, keloids, metastatic tumors.

Brown papules. Nevi, seborrheic keratoses [Figure 2-9], inflamed seborrheic keratosis [Figure 2-10], dermatofibroma, malignant melanoma.

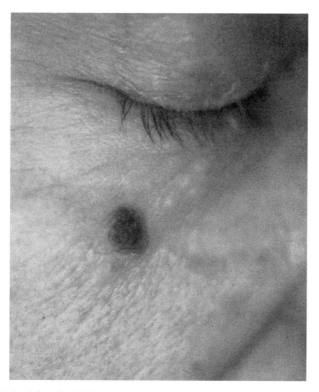

Figure 2-9. Seborrheic Keratosis
These are probably the most common lesions that are seen in patients as they age. They appear as papules and nodules and are often hyperkeratotic. Occasionally also considered to have a greasy quality. Patients often present because of concern that a new keratosis represents melanoma.

Diagnosis

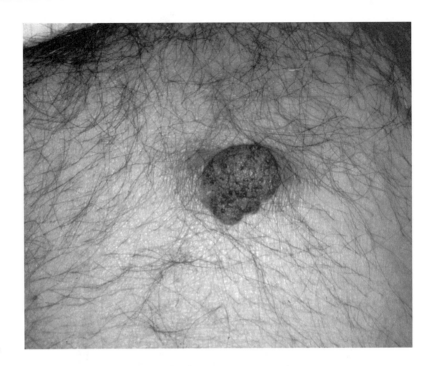

Figure 2-10. Inflamed Seborrheic Keratosis
This inflamed keratosis is benign but patients present with complaints of discomfort.

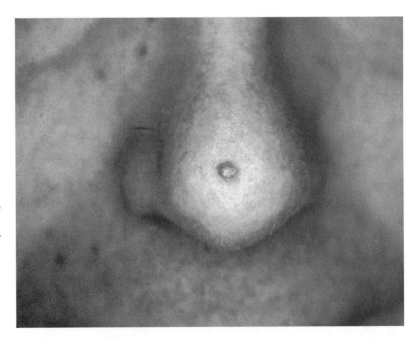

Figure 2-11. Blue Nevus
This nevus is characterized by a bluish color. This lesion highlights the fact that the color of lesions is dependent on how deep in the skin the cells are located. The deeper the pigment is within the dermis, the more blue the lesion will appear because of the Tyndall effect.

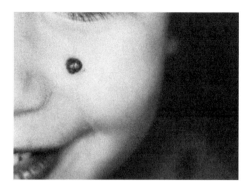

Figure 2-12. Hemangioma
This is a red nodule on the face of a young child. It represents a hemangioma and is similar in appearance to a pyogenic granuloma, another common lesion in childhood.

Blue/black papules. Blue nevus [Figure 2-11], giant comedone, foreign-body, malignant melanoma.

NODULE. A bump on the skin usually considered to be 1 centimeter or larger with extension into the dermis and which can be perceived by palpation.

Red nodules. Angioma, hemangioma [Figure 2-12], Kaposi's sarcoma.

CRUST. Commonly referred to as a scab. Consists of a combination of dried serum and adherent horny cells. May also contain other dried components of wound or lesional exudate.

BLISTER. An elevation of the skin at the dermal/epidermal junction; may be any size. Usually filled with clear fluid.

VESICLE. A small blister.

PUSTULE. A vesicle filled with pus. Appears as a white, cone-shaped papule [Figure 2-13].

CYST. A nodule situated within the deep dermis or subcutis. Usually fluid filled.

EROSION. An area of any size in which the epithelium has been lost through disease or removed by trauma.

ULCER. An area of complete loss of epithelium extending into the dermis.

Diagnosis

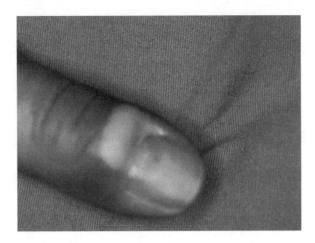

Figure 2-13. Pustules
The pustule is a sign of infection and consists of a collection of white blood cells and other debris within the top layer of the skin such that a small blister forms. In this case, the infection represents a paronychia which must be incised and drained.

ATROPHY.   A loss or diminution of the epidermis, dermis, or other tissue such that a concavity may be appreciated.

ERYTHEMA.   Redness.

STUDYING THE LESION

To properly study any skin lesion, good lighting and a few simple instruments are required. The light should be natural, but when this is not possible an incandescent source is preferable to fluorescent lighting. The ability to illuminate a lesion from the side helps evaluate whether or not a lesion is elevated, so a flashlight is very helpful. Transillumination of lesions by very intense light can help determine whether a lesion is cystic. A Wood's light or black light, which emits in the ultraviolet range, can localize the presence of melanin in the epidermis. Melanin, the common tanning pigment in skin, strongly absorbs at 360 nanometers. Loss of melanin not visible to the naked eye can be highlighted by the use of the Wood's lamp. Hypopigmented areas appear as pale white, and depigmented areas are totally achromatic. On the other hand, subtle pigmentation representing extension of lentigo maligna may be detected with the Wood's lamp and help define the correct margins for excision.

A magnifying glass is the most important tool a dermatologist carries. It should have the capacity to magnify at 5× to 10×. In a pinch, the lens from an ophthalmoscope can be removed and used as an independent magnifier. A glass slide may be used to compress the lesion to determine whether or not it has a vascular component. If a lesion blanches on compression, it is probably vascular. However, if the color cannot be eliminated, a granulomatous process may be represented by the yellow-brown discoloration that is present.

COMMON SKIN LESIONS

The techniques of biopsy and excisional surgery described in this book are used routinely in the diagnosis and management of common skin lesions. A description of these lesions and comments about management follow.

Skin Cancers and Precancerous Lesions

Actinic Keratoses

Actinic keratoses are precancerous skin lesions that present on sun-exposed areas [Figure 2-14]. They most commonly present on the face, tops of the ears, and backs of the hands in individuals who are fair skinned and who have spent an extensive period of time in

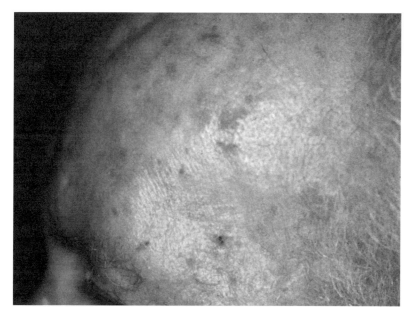

Figure 2-14. Actinic Keratoses
These are multiple small papules that are erythematous and occasionally hyperkeratotic. They are precancerous lesions and are due to sun exposure.

Diagnosis

the sun. Actinic keratoses demonstrate a range of clinical presentations. The most common feature is a rough surface. They may vary from 2–3 mm erythematous macules to hyperkeratotic papules that have a rough, horny surface. Actinic keratoses may also appear as rather large lesions that resemble, and must be distinguished from, squamous cell carcinoma. Treatment approaches include cryosurgery, electrodesiccation and curettage, excision, and topical medical therapies such as 5-fluorouracil.

Basal Cell Cancer

Basal cell cancer is thought to affect over 2 million people a year worldwide and is the most common cancer in humans. There are many clinical subtypes of basal cell cancer, including superficial, cystic, morpheaform, aggressive growth [Figure 2-15], nodular [Figure 2-16], and the classic rodent ulcer [Figure 2-17]. Each of these lesions is relatively easy to identify but must be confirmed by biopsy. Biopsy technique will depend on the suspected depth of the lesion. Treatment options include electrodesiccation and curettage, conventional excision, cryosurgery, and irradiation. Mohs' (microscopically controlled fresh-tissue) excision is especially effective for treating recurrent tumors or those in which one wants to preserve cosmesis and obtain the highest cure rate. Radiation therapy is an option for patients in whom surgery is contraindicated.

Basal cell cancer has a very low metastatic rate but is locally destructive. With each recurrence it tends to become more invasive and difficult to eradicate, so it is preferable to elect a treatment

Figure 2-15a. Aggressive Growth Basal Carcinoma This basal cell carcinoma is far more ominous than it appears on the surface. It has multiple digitate growths that extend within the depth of the dermis and occasionally into the subcutis. *2-15b.* The histologic extent of morpheaform or aggressive growth basal cell cancer can be significantly greater than the clinical appearance on the surface.

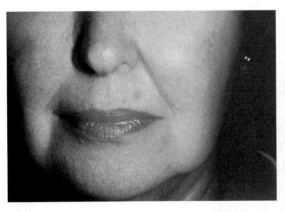
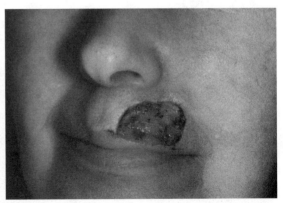

(a) (b)

Common Skin Lesions

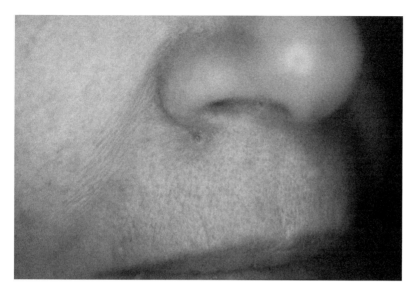

Figure 2-16. Nodular Basal Cell Carcinoma
This classical lesion is a nodule consisting of fine telangiectasias and a pearly surface. Often, a surface erosion will be present and the patient will complain about sporadic bleeding.

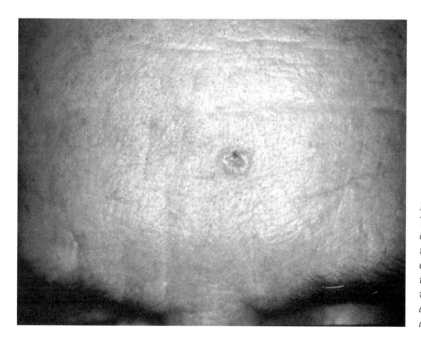

Figure 2-17. Rodent Ulcer
This lesion is a classic basal cell carcinoma, bearing the so-called moniker of rodent ulcer, a term originally used in England in the eighteenth century. They were considered to have the appearance of having been eaten away by a rat.

Diagnosis

approach for the primary lesion that has the highest chance of success.

Squamous Cell Cancer

Squamous cell cancer of the skin is due almost exclusively to ultraviolet radiation. The lesions appear on the head and neck and back of the hands [Figure 2-18]. They are especially problematic in immune-suppressed individuals, such as renal transplant patients, who may die from metastatic disease. The metastatic risk of squamous cell carcinoma is greatest when it occurs on the ears and lips.

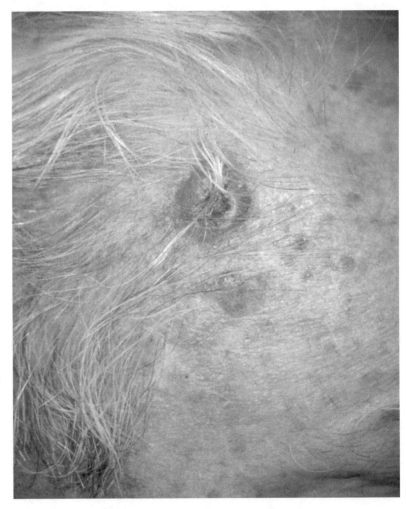

Figure 2-18. Squamous Cell Cancer
This is the more concerning tumor of the class known as nonmelanoma skin cancer. It is a good example of a nodule with a surface ulcer or crater. Note that inferior to it is a hyperkeratotic papule representing an actinic keratosis. Multiple solar lentigos are present as well which indicate chronic sun exposure.

Lentigo Maligna

Lentigo maligna is, in essence, melanoma in situ. Atypical melanocytes percolate throughout the epidermis but there is no invasion into the dermis. Typical lentigo maligna presents as a variegated brownish patch on the face of an older individual [Figure 2-19]. Change in color, shape or size may be noted at some point, which prompts evaluation by biopsy. As the lesions may be very large, biopsy must either be performed in multiple areas, in the darkest area (which is likely to correspond to the deepest part of the lesion), or an incisional biopsy should be done that samples the greatest amount of the lesion. Because lentigo maligna most commonly occurs on the face, this procedure is not always feasible, so a careful strategy aimed at making a determination about the invasiveness of the lesion is indicated.

Melanoma

Melanoma is the most lethal form of skin cancer. It is the one disease that can and should be diagnosed by the primary-care physician in its earliest stages. The characteristic findings are asymmetry, irregular border, variation in color, and relatively large size compared to atypical nevi [Figures 2-20 and 2-21]. Although these features are

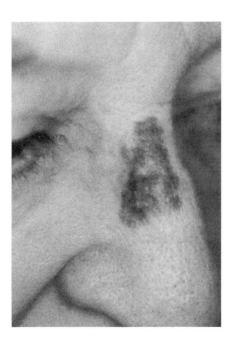

Figure 2-19. Lentigo Maligna
A lentigo maligna presents as a patch of hyperpigmented skin usually on the sun-exposed face of elderly individuals. The lesion represents atypical or malignant cells that are confined to the epidermis and have low invasive potential. However, longstanding lentigo maligna has the potential of developing into lentigo maligna melanoma, which represents the invasive form of disease.

Diagnosis

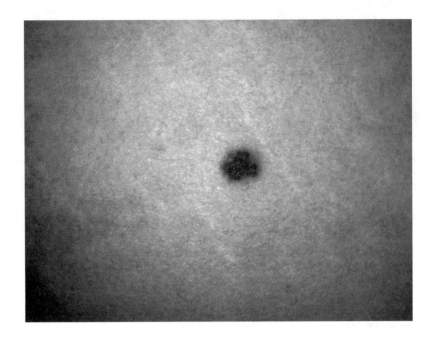

Figure 2-20. Melanoma
This melanoma demonstrates the classic findings of irregularity of contour and color.

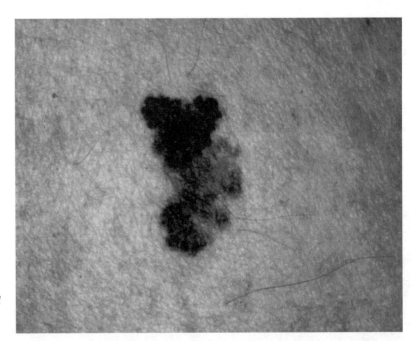

Figure 2-21. Melanoma
Another variant of melanoma characterized by very dark color. Some melanomas are completely black as a result of the melanin pigment that is produced by the cancerous cell. This lesion, although broad, still appears to be clinically in the radial growth phase.

helpful for purposes of public education, they are by no means the sole criteria for the diagnosis of melanoma. The practicing physician should become familiar with melanoma in all of its manifestations and strive to diagnose it at its earliest stage.

True malignant melanoma is easily diagnosed by biopsy. If the patient is already complaining about itching, bleeding, or ulceration, the lesion is more advanced than usual and is at greater risk for metastasis. Unfortunately, although the classic descriptions of melanoma are those that present most commonly in the physician's office, *amelanotic melanoma* exists. In addition, amelanotic lentigo maligna has been reported. Incompletely treated lentigo maligna may lead to *desmoplastic melanoma,* which is a spindle cell tumor. Desmoplastic melanoma demonstrates an increased risk of metastasis and is difficult to eradicate.

Nevi

Nevi, or moles, can represent a challenging routine diagnostic problem for the dermatologist and nondermatologist alike. Over the past several years it has become clear that certain nevi are atypical and either are a red flag that the patient is at risk for developing malignant melanoma or the atypical nevus itself may transform into this lethal skin cancer [Figures 2-22 and 2-23]. It is important to remember that the majority of nevi are completely benign and pose no risk for development into malignant melanoma.

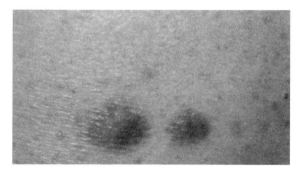

Figure 2-22. Atypical Nevus
An atypical nevus must be distinguished from a normal nevus and a melanoma. Usually an atypical nevus has features that consist of irregularity in contour and in pigmentation. An atypical nevus may represent a lesion that is at risk for turning into a melanoma or be a sign that the patient may be at risk for developing melanoma.

Diagnosis

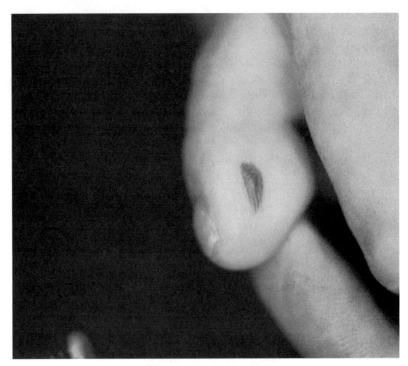

Figure 2-23. Atypical Nevus
Another variant of atypical nevus. Previously, atypical nevi were referred to as dysplastic nevi, but this term has been dropped in favor of the more precise "atypical nevus". The histologic features of the lesion must be considered before a firm diagnosis of atypical nevus can be made.

The cell of origin in the nevus is derived from the neural crest and the first nevus may appear at 6–12 months of age. New lesions continue to develop over time. The average adult Caucasian has approximately 20 to 40 moles [Figure 2-24]. Atypical nevi tend to be seen in families and for this reason present an opportunity for longitudinal follow-up. An individual in whom melanoma has been identified should have all family members evaluated for atypical nevi and melanoma.

An atypical nevus can be identified by a variety of features, but most commonly irregularity, size, and variation in color are the characteristics that define a clinically atypical nevus. In the advanced form, an atypial nevus may well be indistinguishable from a melanoma and for this reason alone would invite biopsy. Once a physician becomes sufficiently comfortable with atypical nevi, it may be possible to monitor them closely either with the aid of photographs or with detailed documentation.

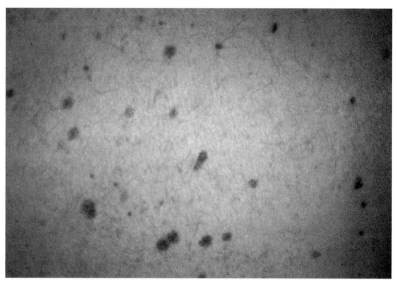

Figure 2-24.
Patients with multiple nevi should be followed by a dermatologist. Distinguishing which nevi are completely benign and which require excision should be based on a thorough clinical appraisal of the lesion. Needless excision of bland or benign nevi should be assiduously avoided.

The atypicality of the nevus in an individual must be viewed within the context of the patient's overall skin examination. An individual who is fair skinned and has freckles and no other nevi except the one under suspicion should probably have it biopsied since it represents a deviation from the norm for that particular patient. Alternatively, an individual who has multiple odd-appearing nevi may be followed closely as those particular nevi may represent the baseline for that person. It may be beneficial, in this case, to biopsy the two or three most abnormal-appearing nevi. If they appear sufficiently bland microscopically, then careful monitoring alone is acceptable.

Patients with atypical nevi have been studied and it has been shown that even if all atypical nevi are completely excised, the risk of developing melanoma does not decrease. It is this observation that suggests atypical nevi may actually serve as a warning that the individual is at risk for melanoma rather than that the specific lesion is at risk for transforming into melanoma itself.

Common Benign Lesions

Sebaceous Hyperplasia

Lesions of sebaceous hyperplasia represent proliferation of the sebaceous glands normally found within the dermis in association with hair follicles. Although this problem is more prominent in men, it can be seen in women. The disorder is easily identified by the central depression within the papule, and the yellowish raised donut-shaped periphery which represents the hyperplasia of the sebaceous unit. Treatment of these lesions is relatively difficult if one wants to be certain to avoid scarring.

Seborrheic Keratoses

Seborrheic keratoses are probably the most common skin lesions in the older population. They present as papules ranging in size from a few millimeters to several centimeters. They have a hyperkeratotic, uneven surface and variegated color. Seborrheic keratoses can sometimes simulate malignant melanoma and often are biopsied for this reason. However, these benign lesions represent a proliferation of epidermal cells that tend not to recur when removed and yield an excellent cosmetic result. They are treated by cryosurgery, electrodesiccation and curettage, or curettage alone. Some dermatologists refuse to treat with cryosurgery because of the risk that the lesion may be a melanoma and failure to obtain tissue for biopsy will preclude a correct diagnosis and proper therapy.

Full thickness excision of seborrheic keratoses is common in certain parts of the country where failure to have a complete clinical understanding of the lesion leads to the mistaken impression that one is dealing with a malignant lesion for which an excisional biopsy is indicated. The distinction of seborrheic keratosis from malignant melanoma is relatively easy to make based on a thorough understanding of the clinical appearance of the lesion. When examined carefully, it is clear that a seborrheic keratosis appears to develop on the surface of the skin, whereas a melanoma, even the superficial spreading type, develops within the top layers of the skin. Magnified examination with good illumination at the periphery of the lesion usually is sufficient to distinguish a seborrheic keratosis from a malignant melanoma. In addition, the verrucous surface of seborrheic keratosis is helpful in this regard. A rare entity in which seborrheic keratosis is not so easily distinguished from melanoma is verrucous melanoma. This lesion, often located on the lower extremity, simulates a seborrheic keratosis but is in fact a melanoma—and of course must be biopsied and diagnosed correctly.

Skin Tags

Skin tags are among the most common skin lesion that you will see in practice. They usually tend to occur around the neck and in the axilla. Patients will present because of cosmetic concerns and because strangulated lesions may start to bleed. Occasionally a strangulated skin tag will appear black and the patient will present concerned about malignant melanoma. A biopsy will rule out this diagnosis. Skin tags are easily excised without local anesthesia, as the instillation of local anesthesia tends to be more painful than the scissor snip itself. A Gradle scissors is recommended but the lesion may similarly be elevated on its stalk by forceps and severed with a scalpel.

There is some debate about the need to send skin tags for pathologic evaluation. Because there are often so many lesions and patients request treatment of most of the lesions at one time, it may appear impractical to send all specimens for dermatopathology. You must make an independent decision based on your certainty of the clinical diagnosis. From the point of view of defensive medicine, even though the lesion you remove is benign, if the patient should present with a metastatic skin cancer such as melanoma in the future, it would be difficult for you to prove that you removed a benign lesion without histologic proof.

Solar Lentigo

Solar lentigos are tan to brown macules or patches that appear on sun-exposed areas. They are commonly known as liver spots or age spots. When uniform in color and contour, the lesions are consistent with benign, sun-related lentigos. However, if irregularity is present in pigmentation or contour, or if the lesion has changed over time, the possibility of lentigo maligna or melanoma in situ must be raised. In this case a biopsy is indicated. Lentigo maligna, which may have been present in older patients for more than 15 years, can be quite broad, though still confined to the epidermis and noninvasive. If left untreated, lentigo maligna can evolve into invasive lentigo maligna melanoma.

Diagnosis

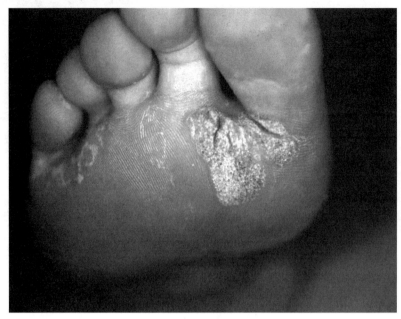

Figure 2-25. Wart
A wart can have a variety of appearances. Figure 2-8 demonstrates condyloma, which are genital warts. However, periungual warts, which are found around the fingernails, and plantar warts have a completely different presentation. They are all caused by the human papilloma virus of which there are more than 60 subtypes.

Warts

Warts are caused by the human papilloma virus of which there are greater than 60 viral subtypes. The condition is especially difficult to treat in its myriad presentations. Common forms include (a) flat warts, which appear as multiple 1–2 mm facial papules in children; (2) periungual warts, which occur as persistent warts in the nail folds of the fingers. When present for a long period of time, squamous cell carcinoma in situ may develop. This form of skin cancer, also known as Bowen's disease, is not invasive; (3) Warts on the palms and soles, which are especially difficult to treat. Surgical approaches may result in permanent scarring and should be carefully considered [Figure 2-25]. In many cases warts will resolve spontaneously. In immune-suppressed patients, however, warts can become a significant problem and challenge even the most skilled dermatologists. In children, Tagamet 300 mg four times a day may speed the natural resolution of warts. Superficial treatments such as cryosurgery or application of caustic agents (bichloracetic acid) may be helpful.

Condyloma

Approximately 30% of the sexually active adult population may carry the human papilloma virus that causes genital warts. The lesions can present as multiple small papules on the shaft of the penis [see Figure 2-8]. When a male is diagnosed with the disease, his sexual partner should also be examined for cervical lesions. Squamous cell carcinoma of the cervix has been associated with genital condyloma. Treatment approaches can include cryosurgery, electrodesiccation and curettage, excision, and laser. However, topical therapy such as podophyllin extract may be successful.

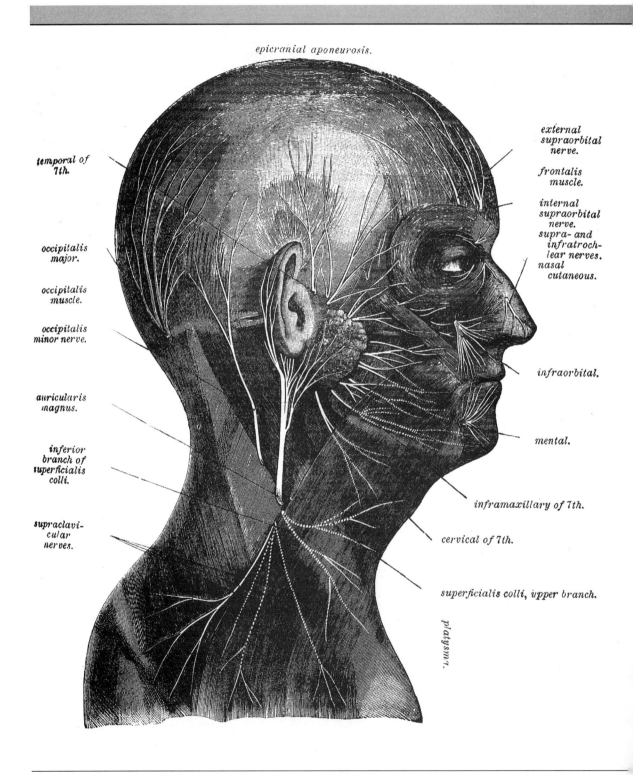

3

Practical Anatomy

The integument, popularly known as the skin, covers a surface area of 3.73 square meters in the average adult. It is the body's largest organ and, in essence, serves to contain all others. The skin is also the most extensive sensory organ and as such subsumes the tasks of pain sensation, eroticism, and defense. It dynamically monitors ambient and internal temperature and tightly regulates fluctuations that might otherwise interfere with normal physiologic processes. Its intrinsic anatomical qualities include flexibility of a degree that has never been duplicated by any synthetic material.

In the Middle Ages, chain mail was a crude attempt at accommodating the need of the body's extremities to flex and extend during battle. The search for a "second skin" has continued into modern times, but even material as remarkable as latex is nonregenerative and will eventually wear out. The skin, however, provides what no polymer can: the ability to repair and regenerate. Take a moment to look at your knee: bend it. Notice how the skin over the joint expands to accommodate the significant expansion of surface area created by the flexion of the joint. Similarly, consider the extent to which your mouth deforms during conversation and while eating (though, one hopes, not by doing both at the same time).

The remarkable elastic capacity of the skin to accommodate deformation is matched or exceeded by the physiological dynamic known as wound healing. This exceedingly complex (and not fully understood) process by which the skin recovers from injury, accidental or intended, makes it a truly remarkable organ. We are endowed with two eyes, an oversized liver, two kidneys, an exceedingly long gut, 10 toes, 10 fingers, and a host of other duplicated tissue, in part because of the reality that through the rough and tumble of chasing down food, seeking out shelter, and fending off invaders of our space, both human and microbial, we will, at one time or another, suffer attrition of our various parts and components. While the skin itself does not wholly duplicate itself when injured, it does bear a remarkable ability to regenerate in other ways. It is the anatomy of the skin that at once accommodates its self-regeneration and permits its repair by human hands.

A thorough understanding of the anatomy of the skin, both microscopic and regional, is critical to successful dermatologic surgery. Procedures as simple as a biopsy require a knowledge of the histology and regional skin tension forces. Because of the largely cosmetic nature of many of the procedures that are performed in dermatology, biopsy techniques that minimize scarring will be appreciated by the patient. While the traditional methods of full-thickness excision are routinely used by those trained exclusively in plastic surgery, special knowledge of skin anatomy has permitted dermatologists to develop a range of biopsy methods that minimize scarring.

When the skin is violated, a scar will result, regardless of the surgical method used. It is important to understand that patients' perception of the word *scar* is very different from the intended meaning when used by physicians. Most patients believe that scar refers to an unsightly failure to heal properly. Physicians, of course, understand that a scar is a technical term describing the repaired tissue at the site of a previous injury, iatrogenic or otherwise. The issue for the patient should not be whether a scar will result. It often will. What is important to emphasize is whether the scar will be noticeable.

We will review only critical anatomy concepts in this chapter. It is assumed the reader is familiar with the anatomy of the head and neck and so we will focus here on special anatomic considerations as they relate to common skin surgery.

RELAXED SKIN TENSION LINES

One of the most common anatomic concepts relating to skin surgery is that of relaxed skin tension lines. Figure 3-1 demonstrates the classical understanding of these relaxed skin tension lines. Because the skin is draped over the body in a fashion that permits mobility, retraction, extension, expansion, and flexion, it is necessary that

Relaxed Skin Tension Lines

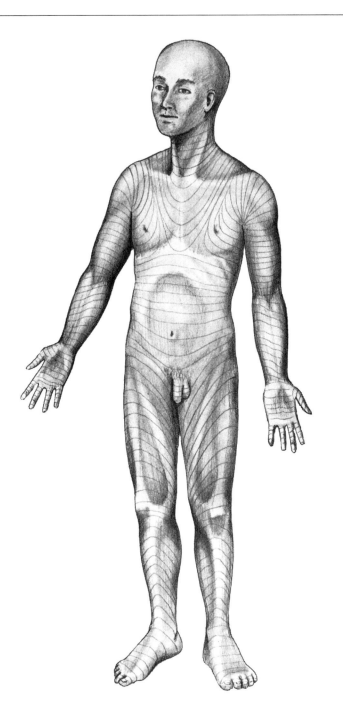

Figure 3-1. Relaxed Skin Tension Lines
The relaxed skin tension lines guide the surgeon in designing the excision to minimize tension on the wound. Although relaxed skin tension lines are generally reliable, it is always necessary for the surgeon to grasp the skin and determine the actual skin tension lines in the individual patient. Reprinted with permission from Bennett, Richard G., 1988, Fundamentals of Cutaneous Surgery, *Mosby, St. Louis, MO, p. 366.*

greater latitude be provided in certain parts of the body than others. For example, because of the necessity for great movement in the mouth region and because of the need for facial expression, the face is endowed both with numerous muscles and excess skin to accommodate the movement of those muscles. Over time, the excess skin conspires with the loss of elastic tissue to create wrinkles and age lines. These lines often reflect the relaxed skin tension lines.

By contrast, the skin over the shoulder is thick and subject to much tension. But even with these factors at play, one can usually find one direction in which the skin can be apposed with the least tension. This represents the relaxed skin tension line and it is normally within these lines and parallel to them that excisions or procedures should be performed. The scheme in Figure 1 simply represents general guidelines. Each individual will demonstrate unique relaxed skin tension lines that should be followed independently of what this or any other text conveys.

REGIONAL CONSIDERATIONS

Mouth

The vertical rhytids seen on the upper and lower lips are easily recognized [Figure 3-2]. They result from the contraction of the orbicularis oris. They are more prominent in smokers and often have a genetic basis. Patients will often tell you that their mother and grandmother had the same problem. Repairs in this area should be done within the relaxed skin tension lines; repairs perpendicular to it will likely result in hypertrophy secondary to the underlying muscle contraction. At times, a linear repair is best done in a counterintuitive fashion. For example, one would expect that a repair hidden in the horizontal forehead creases would be better concealed than a vertical linear closure. In fact, in the central forehead, contraction of the frontalis will often put tension on the horizontal repair and cause it to hypertrophy or contract. A vertical scar has a better chance of healing in a fine, indistinct fashion.

Nose

The muscles of the nose assist in the gentle movement of the nostrils related to breathing. As a result, although one might not normally

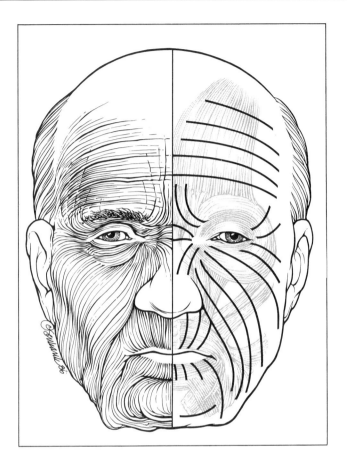

Figure 3-2. Rhytides
Facial rhytides reflect the underlying muscular anatomy of the face. Variations in facial expression must be considered when deciding the proper alignment of a surgical scar within the lines of facial expression. Reprinted with permission from Salasche, S., Bernstein, G., and Senkarik, M., 1988, Surgical Anatomy of the Skin, *Appleton, Norwalk CT, p. 31.*

expect it, there is always a possibility of developing hypertrophic scarring over the alar wings. For this reason, excision and biopsy should be done cautiously.

Ears

The anatomy of the ear is complex and it is important to know the terminology of the subunits [Figure 3-3]. The ears themselves are not prone to any special scarring and repair is remarkably easy because of the very dense vascular supply. Interestingly it is proba-

Practical Anatomy

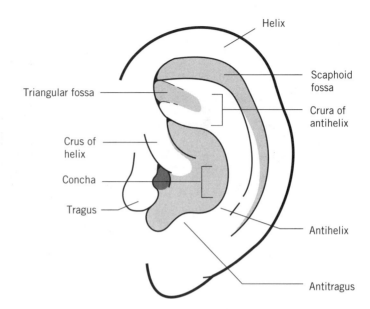

Figure 3-3. Ears
The ear anatomy is complex and it is important to be familiar with each of the subunits as described above.

bly because of the increased vascular supply of the ears and the lymphatic investment of this region that squamous cell carcinoma may have an increased risk of metastasis. The earlobes tend to be an area where hypertrophic scarring and keloiding can form, although the basis for this is not well understood.

Eyes

The eyelids and lips both represent free margins. For purposes of repair, these areas require special care. On the one hand, eyelid margins tend to heal from biopsy very well because of the strong support provided by the tarsus. On the other hand, if the tarsus is violated, healing with a notch is not uncommon. The thin skin of the upper and lower eyelids is a surgeon's dream because healing is often extremely simple with very good cosmetic results. The crow's-feet provide abundant lax skin for repair, although one must always be careful not to violate the lateral canthus, especially in older patients. In this group, senile laxity of the lower lid may predispose to ectropion if the procedure creates downward tension.

Scalp

The scalp is endowed with a very extensive blood supply. As a result, any surgery in this area has the advantage of healing well and the disadvantage of being slowed by the challenge of hemostasis. Suction is often required. Because of the massive collateral circulation on the scalp, and on the face for that matter, it is difficult to compromise the vascular supply during surgery. The underlying galea is truly the supporting structure of the scalp and any excision would do well to include approximation of the galea to prevent spreading of the scar [Figure 3-4]. This is especially the case in younger individuals and/or when the excision overlies the temporalis muscle. An especially vulnerable area for spread scar is the anterior hairline in the temple, probably because of the underlying muscle movement.

Neck

The neck and jaw are especially prone to scarring because of the extensive mobility of the neck. Excisions in this area should be performed along the relaxed skin tension lines as much as possible and adequate undermining should be performed. On the neck, undermining may well go down to the level of the platysma.

Back and Chest

The back and chest are two of the most difficult areas for excision [Figure 3-5]. The extensive tension that is present on any wound created over the shoulders, the middle back, and chest is such that one can expect a spread scar in this location or a hypertrophic scar. The thickness of the skin is especially problematic and the dermis may be many times thicker than what one may be used to when working on the face. Inexperienced individuals, when performing excisions on the back, usually perform an inadequate excision and may fail to go through the complete dermis. This prevents proper apposition of the wound and dehiscence may result. Careful monitoring of the wound in the critical first 6 months is necessary. Any sign of hypertrophic scarring should invite consideration of treatment with intralesional steroids. [See Chapter 12.]

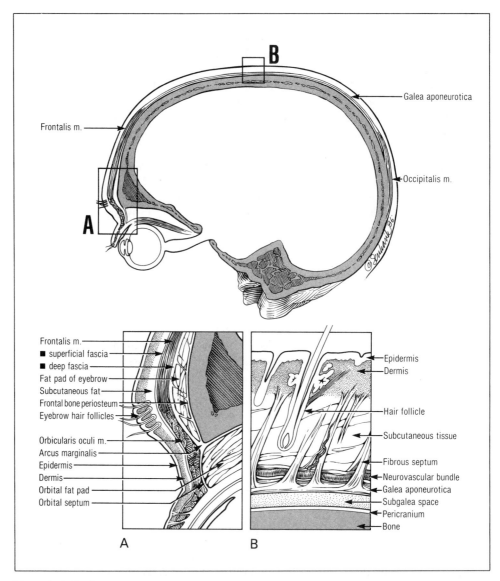

Figure 3-4. Scalp
The anatomy of the scalp. It is important to recognize that the skin is relatively immobile in the temple areas and that the galea aponeurotica extends from the forehead all the way to the nuchal crest. This galea limits the extensibility of the scalp. To increase stretch within the scalp it is sometimes necessary to score the galea. Reprinted with permission from Salasche, S., Bernstein, G., and Senkarik, M., 1988, Surgical Anatomy of the Skin, *Appleton, Norwalk, CT, p. 73.*

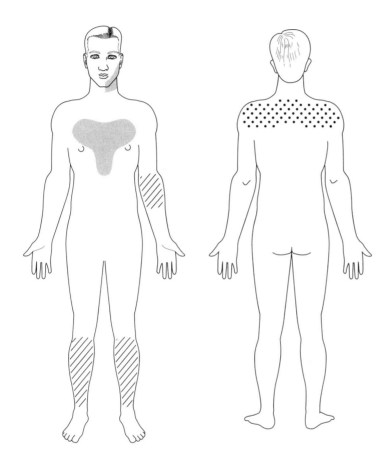

Figure 3-5. Regional Variations
The final cosmetic result of any surgical procedure is often more a result of the location of the excision than the surgical skill of the physician or patient wound care. Certain areas heal poorly whereas others heal well regardless of the technique used.

Upper Extremities

The upper extremity presents a special problem because it is an area of significant tension and movement. In addition, the convexity of the surface often means that a linear excision may lead to puckers. The lazy S fusiform excision described in Chapter 10 helps to resolve this problem. The dorsae of the hands heal well, but the skin tends to be very thin, especially in older individuals. On the other hand, because of the innate mobility of the hands, there is often excessive skin. The vasculature lies within very loose tissue and special attention must be paid when performing an excision in this area. Incision through venous structures is not a problem and often a small ligature is sufficient to control bleeding. Arterial structures are more difficult to injure, but one should always be aware when working on the hand that digital arteries are susceptible to injury.

Lower Extremities

If you can, stay away from the foot. Excisions on the dorsae of the feet can be painful and can take a long time to heal. The general principle is that the further one is away from the heart, the longer it takes for wounds to heal, and this is obvious on the lower extremities. The anterior shin, where it is often difficult to do a linear closure, takes a long time to heal and special approaches are indicated. Although most lesions on the thighs and calves can be closed in a linear fashion, the relatively poor blood supply of the lower extremity will be extremely taxing for advanced repairs such as flaps.

SUPERFICIAL ANATOMY

A detailed review of head and neck anatomy is beyond the scope of this book. We aim, therefore, to provide important information about the superficial anatomy as it relates primarily to your planning and execution of skin surgery on the head and neck. Anatomic issues, such as nerve supply in other regions of the body, are addressed in the chapter on local anesthesia.

The anatomy of the head and neck region is best considered by viewing the face in the Frankfort plane or horizontal frontal view. Generally speaking, the face is divided into three segments in a horizontal plane and five segments in a vertical plane [Figure 3-6]. The superior horizontal segment extends from the hairline to the eyebrows. The middle segment extends from the eyebrows to the upper lip and the third horizontal segment of the face extends from the upper lip to the chin. These roughly equivalent segments help us understand the physical balance of facial structure so that we are able to design our repairs in a manner respectful of them.

The vertical division of the face includes two lateral sections that extend from the ears and preauricular area to the lateral canthus. Two medial central sections of the face extend from the lateral canthus to the medial canthus of the eye; and the central facial region, which corresponds roughly with the embryonic fusion plane, con-

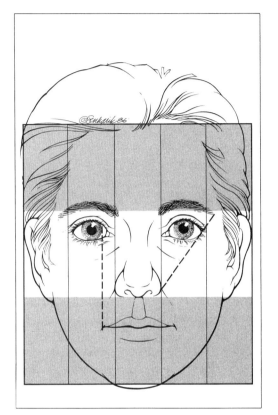 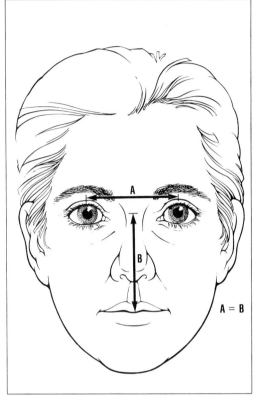

Figure 3-6. Frontal Plane
The frontal plane of the face. It is important when performing surgery on the face to evaluate the patient in the sitting position with the face forward. Reprinted with permission from Salasche, S., Bernstein, G., and Senkarik, M., 1988, Surgical Anatomy of the Skin, *Appleton, Norwalk, CT, p. 31.*

sists of the region defined by the two medial canthi. It happens, by chance, to include the central nose area, the philtrum, and the central chin area.

The face may also be viewed in practical terms with respect to reconstruction. When lesions are removed and repair is performed, it is important to identify areas where excess skin is available. In general, younger patients have skin that is less lax and therefore less available for reconstruction. However, even in patients in their 30s and 40s, reservoirs of additional skin are available in specific regions. After obtaining substantial experience in reconstructing the face, the surgeon will note that he or she naturally views the surface anatomy of the face in the context of what areas can serve to assist in reconstruction. Specifically, Figure 3-7 demonstrates where excess skin is available. It is interesting to note that even in the case of the dorsal aspect of the nose in an older individual who has had substantial sun damage, the cheeks may provide sufficient extra skin for relatively complex reconstructions.

It is best, from a practical point of view, to approach the anatomy of the face in a regional fashion. We have already talked about the mouth and other areas and highlighted issues specific to them. We will focus now on specific anatomic regions and highlight those areas that are at risk for injury during surgery and those that present special problems.

Forehead

The forehead consists of several smaller regions. Near the hairline laterally on both sides the skin is especially immobile, even with undermining. Branches of the temporal artery may be encountered in full-thickness excision in the temple areas and these may require ligature [Figure 3-8]. In addition, transection of branches of the supratrochlear and supraorbital nerves, which are branches of the ophthalmic nerve V_1 may result in spotty numbness of the forehead and scalp for an indefinite period of time [Figure 3-9]. Often this

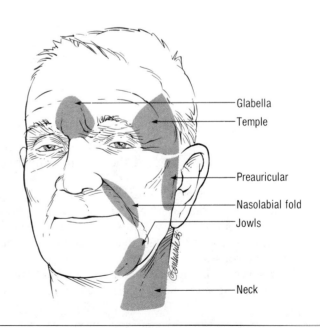

Figure 3-7. Skin Reservoirs When performing surgical repair on the face, it is important to be aware of those areas of excess skin that normally develop with time. These areas often can be mobilized for reconstruction. Reprinted with permission from Salasche, S., Bernstein, G., and Senkarik, M., 1988, Surgical Anatomy of the Skin, Appleton, Norwalk, CT, p. 64.

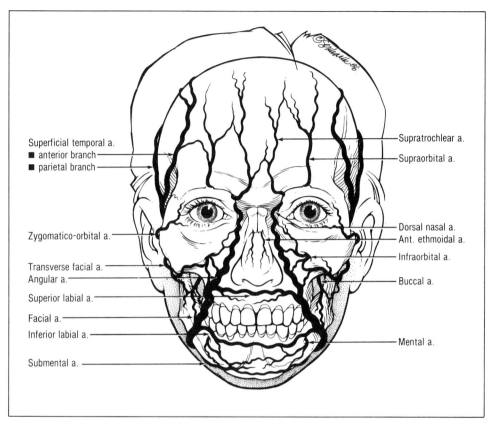

Figure 3-8. Temporal Artery
The temporal artery and associated anatomy is demonstrated above. The face is very well collateralized and ligation of the temporal artery itself rarely results in any significant complication. Reprinted with permission from Salasche, S., Bernstein, G., and Senkarik, M., 1988, Surgical Anatomy of the Skin, *Appleton, Norwalk, CT, p. 130.*

numbness, which can be quite upsetting to patients if they are not warned about it in advance, can last more than 6 months.

When operating on the forehead and scalp, it is important to be cognizant of the fact that injury to hair follicles will result in bald patches. This is especially true when dissecting in the region of the eyebrows and in men this applies to the upper lip and beard area as well. One must always be certain to undermine beneath the level of the hair follicles so that they are not traumatized. The forehead and scalp provide a special measure of safety because of their unique anatomy. Immediately beneath the skin on the forehead is the frontalis muscle. This muscle extends from the region of the eyebrows

Practical Anatomy

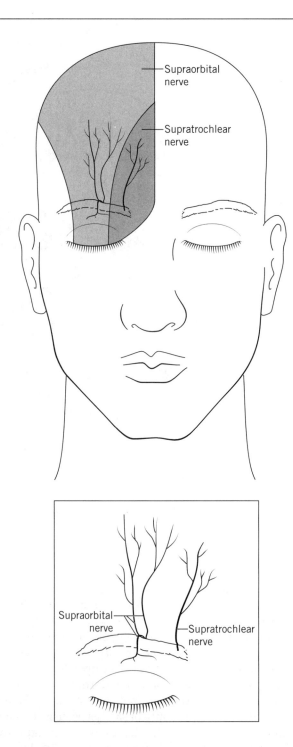

Figure 3-9. The Ophthalmic Nerve
Branches of the ophthalmic nerve. Injury to any of the branches can have a significant effect on sensation.

superiorly and joins with the galea aponeurotica posteriorly. The galea eventually merges into the occipitalis muscle.

Frontally, beneath the frontalis muscle is the deep fascia, which provides a level of safety for dissection. One can dissect back relatively far in a bloodless plane [Figure 3-5]. Over the temple area, the temporalis muscle is a massive structure which, through routine contraction, can lead to a spread scar over time regardless of the success of the original closure. It is in the temple region that one encounters the nerve most commonly injured during routine skin surgery that has the greatest impact on the patient.

Normally, because of the collateralization of vascular structures and nerves, injury to any one branch is not a matter of concern. However, where the temporal nerve crosses the midzygomatic arch, it is at great risk for injury [Figure 3-10]. Both this nerve and the

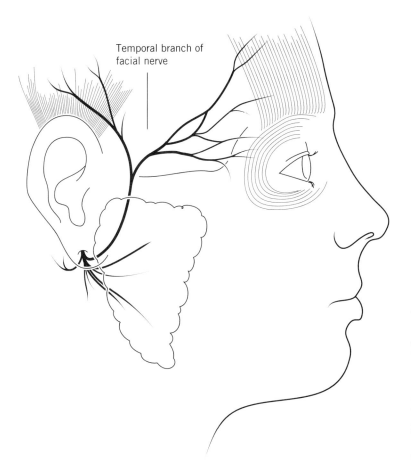

Figure 3-10. Temporal Nerve
The temporal branch of the facial nerve is probably the most commonly injured motor nerve in facial dermatologic surgery because of its superficial location. Trauma to this nerve may result in a lid droop and paralysis of the forehead with loss of the horizontal lines of expression.

marginal mandibular nerve, which is discussed elsewhere, have a limited number of branches, which happen to be located in a very superficial plane. The temporal branch of the facial nerve supplies the upper orbicularis oculi, the frontalis, and the corrugator supercilia muscles. If a line is drawn from the earlobe to the lateral edge of the eyebrow, and from the tragus to just above and behind the highest forehead crease, the region can be defined in which the temporal branch is at greatest risk of injury. More generally, the nerve is at greatest risk as it traverses the midzygomatic arch. Dissection must be carried out in a very superficial fashion in this area and with blunt instruments only. When you know that you will be working in this area it is important to warn the patient that he or she may suffer permanent, uncorrectable damage. Injury in this area will result in a drooping eyelid and inability to move muscles of the forehead. As a result, there will be loss of the lines and wrinkles on the affected side, resulting in an asymmetric appearance of the forehead. This effect may also be observed in a patient presenting with cancer that has infiltrated the temporal branch of the facial nerve [Figure 3-11].

The facial nerve and its branches that supply the perioral muscles are not normally at risk during routine office skin surgery. The nerve in the lateral cheek lies within the parotid and does not normally extend superficially enough to be at risk. However, it is important to be aware of the fact that the seventh nerve, when injured, can cause a paralysis of the muscles of facial expression on the affected side. This is often noticed during procedures in the region when local anesthesia causes a temporary paralytic effect. It is important

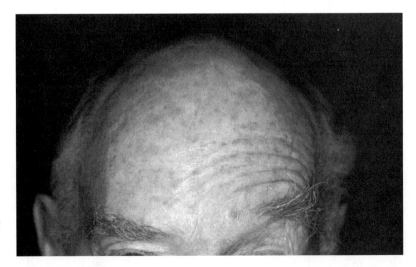

Figure 3-11. Temporal Nerve Injury to the facial nerve or infiltration by tumor may result in paralysis on the ipsilateral side.

Superficial Anatomy

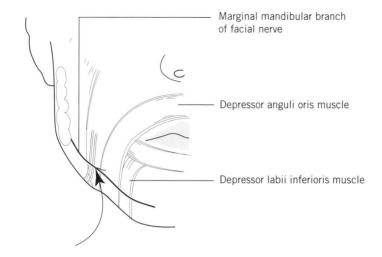

Figure 3-12. Mandibular Nerve Injury
Injury to the mandibular nerve that can occur when operating in the jaw region may result in inability to purse the lip.

to document functioning muscle groups and nerves prior to surgery so that a determination can be made if injury ocurred during the operative procedure. The marginal mandibular nerve supplies the muscles of the mouth and is also a branch of the facial nerve [Figure 3-12]. It is at greatest risk for injury along the jawline and travels with the facial artery. Injury to the marginal mandibular nerve can result in the inability to purse the lips.

Sensory Nerves

The most common sensory nerves that can be injured during facial surgery include the infraorbital nerve [Figure 3-13], which exits the skull in the midpupillary line and supplies the upper lip and nasal sidewall. Although under normal circumstances it is unlikely that one would have to operate at such a deep level, injury to this nerve is conceivable and would be confirmed by paresthesias or numbness in the distribution area. The other sensory nerves include the supraorbital and supratrochlear, already described.

Blood Supply

The face is richly endowed with blood vessels. As mentioned, over the temple area it is quite possible to encounter a larger vessel that is a branch of the temporal artery, which is probably the largest vessel that will be encountered during facial skin surgery. A branch of the labial artery, the angular artery, is often encountered when operating on skin cancers in the nasal alar groove. Similarly, both

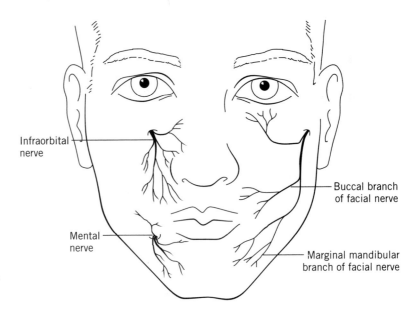

Figure 3-13. Infraorbital Nerve
The infraorbital nerve exits the skull in the midpupillary line. Injury to this nerve will result in loss of sensation to the upper lip and part of the nostril.

the superior and inferior labial arteries, which are branches of the facial artery, may be encountered during lip surgery and are easily ligated or cauterized [Figure 3-14].

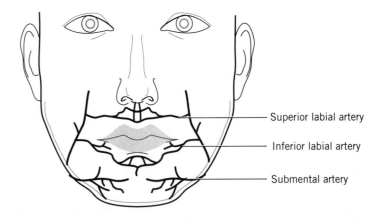

Figure 3-14. Labial Artery
The labial artery supplies both the upper and lower lips. Branches of it extend superiorly and form the angular artery, which is often injured when removing basal cell cancers deep in the alar groove.

Special Considerations in the Neck

The spinal accessory nerve, which controls movement of the scapula, is probably the most vulnerable nerve of the neck region. The spinal

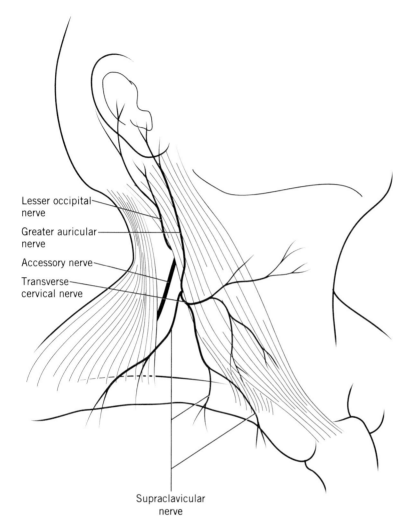

Figure 3-15. Accessory Nerve
The accessory nerve can occasionally be injured while operating on the neck. Trauma to the accessory nerve will result in an inability to lift the scapula.

accessory nerve emerges approximately 2 cm above Erb's point [Figure 3-15]. Erb's point is identified by drawing a line connecting the angle of the mandible with the mastoid process. A vertical line dropped 6 cm from the midpoint of this first line meets the posterior border of the sternocleidomastoid muscle at Erb's point. Wing scapula results from injury to the spinal accesory nerve.

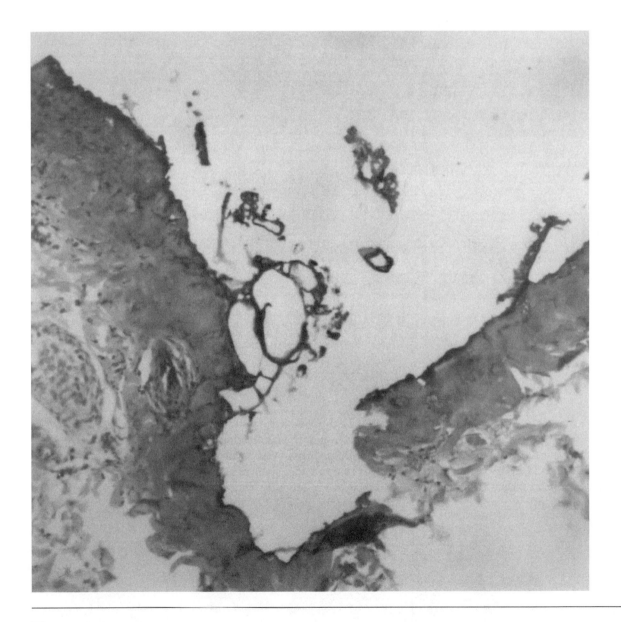

4

Wound Healing

An understanding of wound healing enhances the work of the skin surgeon in the same way that knowledge of Latin improves our use and appreciation of English. The sequence of events that extends from a full-thickness incision of the skin to the mature, remodeled scar is described here as these events underlie the complications that may arise from skin surgery. Understanding the biology, however dry at times, will permit the surgeon to enhance results and minimize complications.

There are three stages in classical wound healing: inflammation, proliferation, and maturation. Wounds can heal either by primary intention wherein the wound edges are approximated and secured by sutures in an artificial fashion, or by delayed second-intention healing. Our approach to wound dressings and care in the latter case is dictated by current knowledge of wound biology.

PHASES

The *inflammatory phase* of wound healing begins at approximately 12 hours after incision, peaks at 36 hours, and is usually resolved by the fifth day. The *proliferative phase* begins shortly after 24 hours, peaks at approximately 8 days, but continues through 45–60 days. The *maturation phase*, which corresponds most directly with wound tensile strength, begins as early as 6 days after surgery, peaks at approximately 2 months, and slowly returns to baseline by 6 months.

Wound Healing

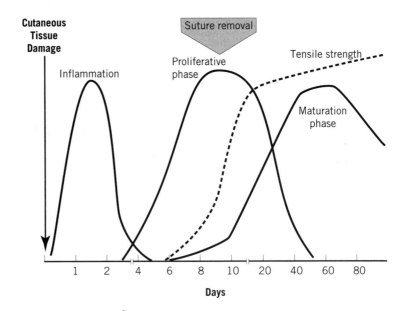

Figure 4-1. Wound Maturation
All skin wounds go through a predictable period of maturation. Wound maturation is not complete until 9–12 months after surgery during which time collagen remodeling continues.

Tensile strength, the factor that determines how strongly a wound will hold, is first apparent at 6 days, continues in a steep incline to approximately 45 days, and increases slowly with the wound maturation process through 1 year [Figure 4-1].

Inflammation

The inflammation stage is initiated with hemorrhage that results from the scalpel incision. In a sense, a wound that does not first bleed does not heal. Adequate blood flow to the wound edges is both an indication of the potential for rapid healing and a source of a panoply of agents that work, domino-like, to culminate in a restored integument. Released proteolytic enzymes activate factor XII, which leads to the inflammation cascade. Important components of this process include the intrinsic coaglation system, the kinin system, the plasminogen-fibrinogen system, and classical complement. Early on, soluble mediators of inflammation transiently increase vascular permeability and facilitate the movement of cellular elements. Neutrophils, platelets, fibroblasts, endothelial cells, and epithelial cells are all important in the response of the skin to injury.

Coagulation, the primary biologic process that makes surgery possible in the first place, is mediated most importantly by platelet activation. The skin surgeon must understand this phase because many medications are commonly prescribed that affect platelet adhesion and activation [Table 4-1]. Failure of platelets to function properly results in abnormal bleeding, which itself can lead to an array of common complications of skin surgery.

The inflammatory response is the body's first molecular attempt at repairing the surgical injury. Specifically, neutrophils and macrophages react with lymphocytes to stimulate fibroblast activity. Platelet-derived growth factor, a protein produced by the activated platelet, is a critical part of the early stage of inflammation and is essential in the initiation of the wound repair process.

Twelve to 36 hours following surgery, neutrophils reduce the bacterial count at the site of incision and minimize local infection. It is important to note that skin infections are very rare under normal circumstances. Unlike internal organ surgery in which there is a cornucopia of potentially hostile bacteria, normal skin flora is nonpathogenic and the robust blood supply of the skin is sufficient to keep the bacterial inoculum to a minimum. The macrophage, derived from the bone marrow and attracted to the wound site by a host of chemotactic factors, assists in minimizing infection and aiding fibroblasts in wound repair. Fibrin, which is a product of the coagulation system, creates a lattice work. The key element of this matrix is the glycoprotein called fibronectin. It is produced by fibroblasts and endothelial cells and, of course, is found in serum. This substance permits the adhesion of cells to a variety of surfaces and is also chemotactic for additional fibroblasts and epithelial cells. Fibroblasts manufacture collagen, which is deposited within the fibronectin-fibrin matrix. By the time collagen predominates in the wound-healing process, fibronectin has disappeared from the wound site.

TABLE 4-1 Systemic Drugs with Inhibitory Effect on Wound Healing

Agent
Actinomycin D
Anticoagulants
Aspirin
Bleomycin
Carmustine
Colchicine
Glucocorticosteroids
Penicillamine
Phenylbutazone

Proliferation

In the second phase of wound healing, proliferation is the central activity. The fibroblast, a motile cigar-shaped cell that plays an important role throughout all stages of wound healing, arrives and replicates. Its myofibrillar activity aids in wound contracture, which is of special importance in second-intention healing. These fibroblasts adhere to fibrin and collagen and begin to form the foundation for the scar tissue that, after the period of maturation, will be permanently in place.

Collagens are a heterogeneous group of molecules, but Type 1 collagen and Type 3 collagen are important in wound healing. Type 1 is the most common form of collagen present in adult skin and it predominates in the dermis. Type 3 collagen, found mainly in fetal tissue, is present initially in dermal wounds but is eventually replaced by Type 1 collagen as the wound ages. Type 4 collagen is

➥ *Wound Care Myths:* Air is good and a scab is a sign of good healing. *Challenge:* Convince your patient that skin wounds heal fastest in a moist environment.

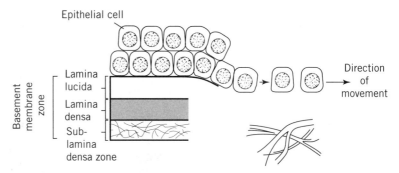

Figure 4-2. Basement Membrane Zone
The complex basement membrane zone is demonstrated here and highlights the fact that there is an integral relationship between the epidermis and the dermis. When the basement membrane zone is not violated in a surgical procedure, scarring will not result. This drawing also demonstrates epithelial migration during the wound healing process. Adapted from Epstein, E. and Epstein, Jr. E., 1987, Skin Surgery, *W. B. Saunders, Philadelphia.*

present in the basement membrane of the skin and is also important in wound healing. Permanent scarring only results if the skin injury violates the basement membrane zone [Figure 4-2]. Techniques described in this book will allow for diagnostic procedures that in many cases protect that zone and permit minimal or no scarring.

Scar

Collagen synthesis is well documented and represents, through the alignment of many smaller subunits, the stepwise manufacture of a complex cablelike structure [Figure 4-3]. Subunits known as tropocollagen polymerize to form the collagen fiber itself. Once collagen fibers have been formed, they are cross-linked by lysyl oxidase to produce mature collagen. Therapeutic agents, however, can interfere with wound healing at a number of stages. For example, penicillamine interferes with the production of mature collagen at this cross-linking stage. Similarly, colchicine blocks the production of collagen at an earlier phase when procollagen is secreted by the fibrocyte. Therefore, it is important to obtain a full drug history.

After the early phases of wound healing, when the collagen has been rebuilt and new epithelium has migrated over the wound base, it is important to focus on the more long-term aspect of the process. The tendency of scars to remodel over time has a corollary in the clinical behavior of the repaired tissue. For example, as the body digests those new collagen fibers that were laid down in a chaotic and nonfunctional fashion, new fibrils are produced that are more

Phases

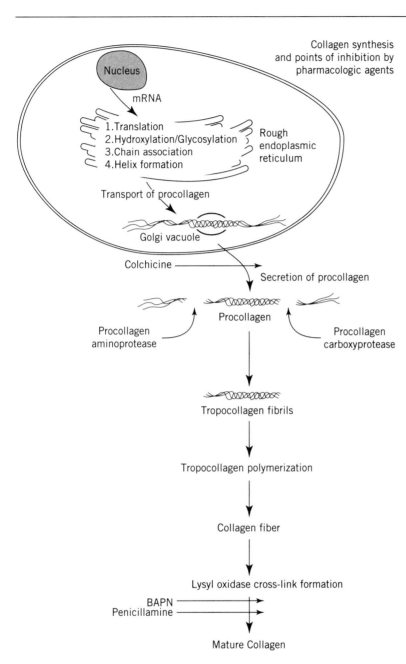

Figure 4-3. Collagen
Collagen production is the physiologic mainstay of wound repair and can be affected by a variety of medications and medical states. The sequential development of the collagen fiber is demonstrated here. Adapted from Epstein, E. and Epstein, Jr. E, 1987, Skin Surgery, W. B. Saunders Co. Philadelphia.

compact and more functional. Analogously, in the first 6 months of tissue repair, the scar tissue engine is in high gear. Perhaps to protect against dehiscence, the scarring mechanism seems to overcompensate. Hypertrophic scars are occasional examples of this. In time, though, the collagen remodeling normalizes the scar, and what was in the early stages a thick, unsightly red bulge of tissue, by 1 year is often flat, if not depressed, and atrophic or white. The maturation process is, in essence, one of balance between the manufacture of collagen and its destruction. While the newly synthesized collagen has very poor wound strength and is more like a gel than a mass of hemp cables, mature collagen is what provides wounds with the breaking strength that characterizes the final wound. Understanding

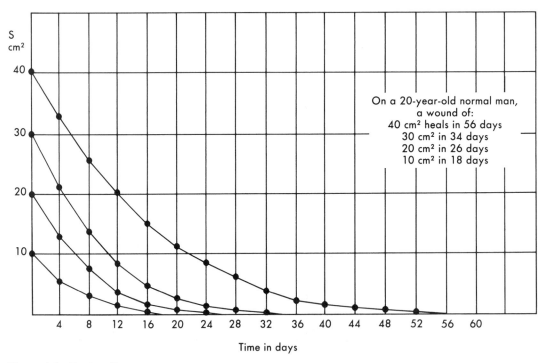

Figure 4-4. Contraction
All skin wounds contract and heal completely on their own if allowed to do so. "Healing by second intention" is often an excellent option when the patient is ill or cannot tolerate more complex reconstructive surgery. Wound contraction is dependent on age, the original size of the wound, and its location. S = surface area. Reprinted with permission from Bennett, R. G., 1988, **Fundamentals of Cutaneous Surgery**, *Mosby, St. Louis, MO.*

the stages at which collagen is remodeled, reformed, and reinvigorated is important to the skin surgeon as he or she considers the method of wound closure.

Second Intention Healing

Often, the ideal wound closure choice is no repair at all. Second-intention healing, a remarkable process of autologous reconstruction, is accomplished primarily by the contractile activity of fibrocytes and myofibroblasts. Such contraction proceeds at approximately 0.75 mm per day [Figure 4-4]. Circular wounds contract more slowly than do rectangular or star-shaped ones. Many factors affect wound healing, and reportedly one of the most important is patient

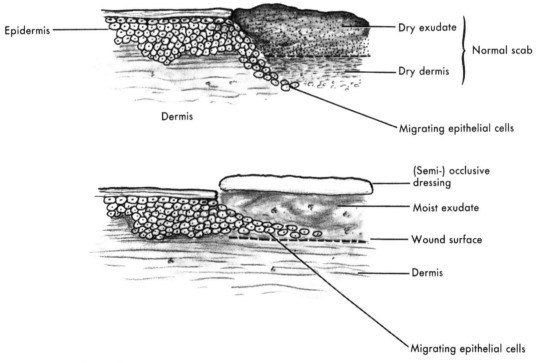

Figure 4-5. Moist Environment
All skin wounds heal best in a moist environment. When wounds are exposed to the air, the cells desiccate and prevent the orderly migration of new epidermal cells into the wound environment. Reprinted with permission from Bennett, R. G., 1988, Fundamentals of Cutaneous Surgery, *Mosby, St. Louis, MO.*

TABLE 4-2 Occlusive Dressings

Dressing	Vendor	Comment
Hydrocolloids		
Duoderm	Convatec	Adheres well.
		Wound fluid becomes soupy and requires drainage.
		Small patches available for biopsy sites
Gels		
Vigilon	Bard Home Health	Gelatinous sheet is packaged between two removable plastic sheets. Both can be removed for complete permeability.
		Minimal oozing
		Best if refrigerated after opening.
		Some adherence to wound
Foams		
Allevyn	Smith & Nephew	Nonadhesive
		Requires additional taping
		Maintains moist environment
Transparent Film		
Tegaderm	3M	Adheres well
		Non-absorbent: maintains fluid in direct contact with wound bed
		Pevents staining of clothes by wound fluid
		Can see wound through it
		Also useful for applying topical medication under occlusion

age. In general, younger patients heal better but have a greater risk of hypertrophic scarring, whereas older patients, especially those with a history of sun exposure, usually have a better opportunity for a cosmetically acceptable scar. Nutritional factors have been cited in wound healing, but none have been identified that, when added to the diet in excess of normal intake or applied topically in a pharmacologic concentration, actually have an impact on the rate of dermal or epithelial healing.

Once the dermis has contracted and regrown with the aid of newly laid-down collagen, attention must turn to epithelial resurfacing. The most important fact to know about epidermal healing is that it proceeds best in a moist environment [Figure 4-5]. When a wound is exposed to the air, the wound bed desiccates and retards further ingrowth of epidermis. The rapid healing of moist wounds (increased healing up to 50%) has been so well documented that a whole range of special occlusive dressings has been developed and is now marketed. Such dressings include polyethylene oxide hydrogel, hydrocolloid particles, and polyurethane film. Each of these types of dressings listed in Table 4-2 has its advantages and disadvantages. Only one example in each category is provided. In general there are many manufacturers of similar products. Listing in Table 4-2 is not intended to endorse one product over another.

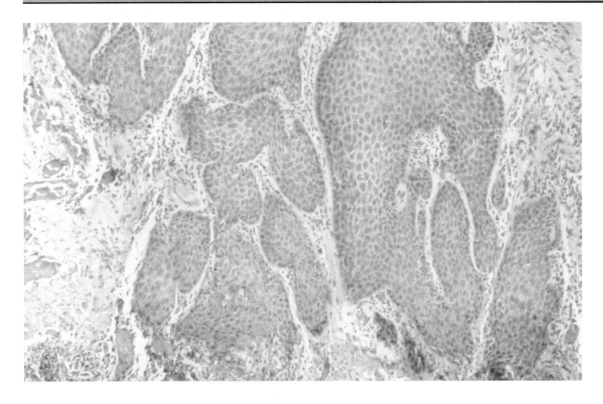

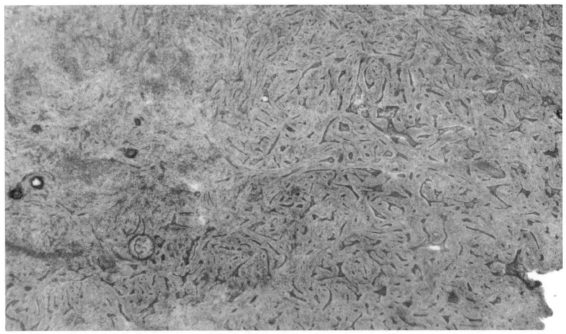

5
Skin Biopsy

A skin biopsy is the removal of a sample of skin and/or underlying soft tissue for purposes of histologic diagnosis. The procedure can be therapeutic (removal of the lesion in its entirety) or diagnostic. It is most commonly performed for the latter purpose to direct therapy or surgical treatment. For example, a suspected basal cell cancer should first be biopsied to establish the diagnosis and histologic subtype (nodular, superficial, infiltrative), so that the appropriate treatment (curettage, excision, Mohs' surgery, etc.) can be recommended. A definitive diagnosis in dermatology can only be made by biopsy of the suspicious tissue.

There are five basic skin biopsy methods: shave, punch, ellipse, scissors excision, and curettage. The technique of choice depends on lesion morphology, location, and cosmetic issues. Inflammatory lesions (e.g., dermatitis) are best sampled with a full-thickness punch biopsy, since a more superficial biopsy may miss pathology evident in the deeper dermis. Likewise, flat or indurated lesions should be biopsied with the punch technique. Elevated, pedunculated, and more superficial lesions (warts, keratoses, acrochordons, nevi) can be sampled with a shave, curette, or scissors technique. A punch biopsy has the advantage of obtaining a specimen deeper into the fat but is limited to the diameter of the punch. A shave biopsy is typically more horizontal than vertical and can obtain a wider, but less deep, specimen. Table 5-1 outlines the advantages and disadvantages of shave and punch biopsies.

Skin Biopsy

TABLE 5-1 Comparison of Shave and Punch Biopsy

	Advantages	Disadvantages
Shave	Rapid (no sutures) Good cosmesis No limit on size of biopsy Can subsequently perform ED&C of skin cancer	Depressed scar if too deep Can't sample deeper soft tissue Can miss deeper component of skin cancer
Punch	Good cosmesis Can sample deeper tissue (into fat) Quicker healing when sutured	Usually requires suturing with sterile technique Limited size Larger punch (5 or 6 mm) can leave dog-ear deformity Cannot subsequently perform ED&C of skin cancer Depth of biopsy limited to length of cylinder

INCISIONAL VERSUS EXCISIONAL BIOPSY

Biopsy procedures are either incisional (remove only part of the lesion) or excisional (remove the lesion in its entirety) [Figure 5-1]. A punch biopsy may be excisional if it removes the entire lesion (e.g., punch excision of a 3 mm nevus) or incisional if it is only a partial sample of a larger lesion (e.g., 4 mm punch biopsy of a 3 cm lentigo maligna). Likewise, a shave biopsy can remove the entire lesion (excisional) or only a part of it (incisional) [Table 5-1]. As a general rule, if the entire lesion can be removed with the biopsy procedure, assuming acceptable cosmesis and healing, it is desirable

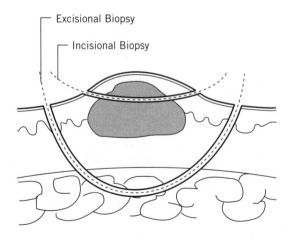

Figure 5-1. Incisional vs. Excisional Biopsy
Incisional biopsy involves removal of part of the lesion while an excisional biopsy implies that the complete lesion is removed by this procedure.

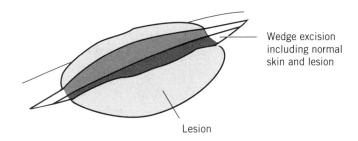

Figure 5-2. Wedge Biopsy
Wedge biopsy permits removal of part of the pathologic tissue as well as normal skin for purposes of comparison.

to do so. It is always critical to provide the pathologist with an adequate specimen for diagnosis.

At times it may be advantageous for the pathologist to view adjacent normal skin along with the skin lesion or pathologic specimen. This procedure is referred to as a wedge excision and can provide a larger and deeper specimen. It may be required for more complex skin diseases, such as a deep panniculitis, deep skin ulcerations (pyoderma gangrenosum), cutaneous lymphoma, or atypical infections [Figure 5-2].

It is a matter of debate whether to remove possible skin cancers by shave or punch biopsy. The advantage of a shave biopsy is that it leaves behind a firm, unaffected dermis upon which one can later perform a definitive procedure such as electrodesiccation and curettage (ED&C). Because a punch biopsy will create a full-thickness defect, it makes subsequent therapy with ED&C more difficult to perform and may result in less satisfactory cosmesis. A shave biopsy has the associated risk of missing evidence of deeper infiltration or invasion by a skin cancer or other pathologic process. A common example of this problem is the biopsy of a suspected squamous cell carcinoma. The pathologist reports in situ Bowen's disease but with the stipulation, "Because the lesion extends to the base of the biopsy specimen, a deeper invasive squamous cell carcinoma cannot be ruled out." A punch biopsy would have provided the base of the lesion and possible evidence of deeper invasion. Likewise, a biopsy of a suspected basal cell carcinoma, if superficial, may miss evidence of deeper infiltrative strands of the carcinoma. Clinical judgment, therefore, is often necessary to select the proper biopsy technique.

SHAVE BIOPSY

The shave biopsy is a quick and easy method of removing superficial lesions. It is more rapid than a punch biopsy because suturing or

Skin Biopsy

other involved methods of hemostatis are usually not required. The shave biopsy can provide a larger and wider specimen than a punch biopsy, but typically does not sample tissue as deeply. While a punch biopsy can obtain tissue as deep as the fat, a shave biopsy usually extends only into the dermis. Depending on the manipulation of the skin at the time of the shave biopsy and the thickness of the skin at the biopsy site, subcutis can be obtained by the shave technique as well. The more superficial a shave, the quicker the healing and the better the cosmesis.

Deeper shave biopsies can result in a permanent depression in the healed skin. The shave biopsy is ideal for raised lesions confined to the epidermis and superficial dermis. Atypical-appearing melano-

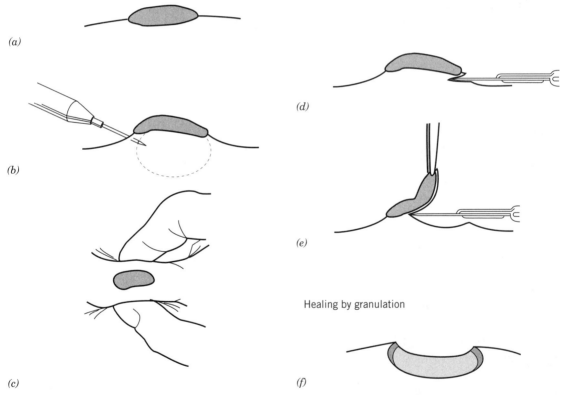

Figure 5-3. Shave Biopsy
A shave biopsy is an excellent method to sample pathologic lesions that are not thought to extend deep into the dermis. The proper method is demonstrated in 5-3a–f. The skin is grasped between fingers. A scalpel or razor blade is then used in a sawing motion across the lesion attempting to keep it flush with the surrounding skin. After the sample has been removed, it is carefully placed in the pathology specimen bottle. The area is either cauterized or hemostasis is obtained with aluminum chloride (Drysol).

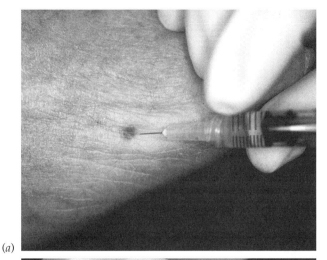

(a)

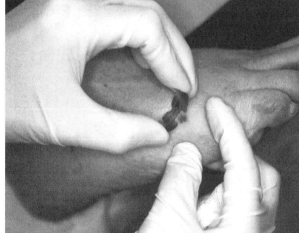

(b)

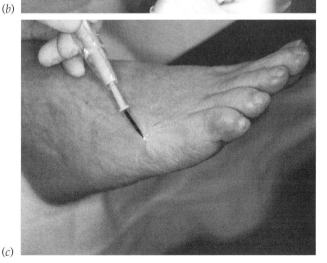

(c)

Shave Biopsy with Razor Blade

(a) Infiltrate the lesion with anesthetic to raise a bleb under it. A 30-gauge 1/2 inch needle is ideal.

(b) Grasp the razor blade between thumb and forefinger while applying lateral traction with your other hand. Gently advance the blade in a sawing motion with nominal side-to-side movement. Adjust the arc of the blade to the curvature and texture of the skin.

(c) Obtain hemostasis with electrocautery or aluminum chloride.

cytic lesions should *not* be removed with the shave procedure unless one is actually going to perform a tangential excision that is certain to include the base of the lesion.

The shave biopsy is usually performed with either a No. 15 Bard Parker blade or a sterilized razor blade [Figure 5-3]. One of the authors (DJL) prefers the latter and uses them almost exclusively because they are extremely sharp, flexible, and inexpensive. The Gillette Blue Blade is attractive because of its carbon steel blade. The razor blade can be gently curved to match the surface upon which the lesion sits. The blade, held by thumb and forefinger at either end, is then advanced across the base of the lesion with a steady, back-and-forth sawing motion. The series of photographs on page 65 show an actual shave biopsy.

The specific steps for use of a scalpel blade or razor blade for biopsy are outlined as follows:

1. The skin may be cleaned with 70% isopropyl alcohol, Betadine, or chlorhexidine. It is true that alcohol prep has never been shown to decrease the risk of infection. In fact, because the biopsy site is exposed and resident skin flora are always present, it is not clear that any particular prep at the biopsy site has a substantial impact.

2. Local anesthesia is achieved with a 30 gauge needle and a 1 cc syringe. A small wheal is raised under the lesion to facilitate the shave biopsy and to keep it superficial [Figure 5-3*b*].

3. The skin is immobilized by stretching it between the thumb and index finger or by pinching it into a more raised position [Figure 5-3*c*].

4. The blade is brought through the base of the lesion in a back-and-forth manner or by pulling through in one direction and then repeating the process until the lesion is excised completely [Figure 5-3*d*]. Forceps can be used to gently pick up the edge of the lesion and provide upward traction, thus allowing visualization of the base of the lesion [Figure 5-3*e*].

5. The depth of the shave is controlled by the angle of the blade. The greater the angle, the deeper the shave. Keeping the blade horizontal with the skin surface will ensure a superficial shave specimen.

6. At times, remnants of the lesion will be noted on the edge. These may be easily removed with curettage, scraping with the belly of the #15 blade, or simulating a curette by bending the razor blade and gently curetting the edge of the residual lesion.

TABLE 5-2 Hemostasis for Skin Biopsies

1. Direct pressure and compressive dressings
2. Electrosurgery
3. Chemical agents
   A. Aluminum chloride (20–40%)
   B. Monsel's solution
   C. Silver nitrate sticks
   D. Phenol
   E. Dichloracetic and trichloracetic acid
4. Physiologic agents
   A. Gelatin foam/sponge (Gelfoam)
   B. Oxidized cellulose (Oxycel, Surgicel)
   C. Thrombin
   D. Mirofibrillar bovine collagen (Avitene, Instat)

7. Hemostasis is achieved with pressure, electrosurgical techniques, or chemical cautery. See Figure 5-3f [Table 5-2]. Aluminum chloride is the most popular chemical agent (20–40%) and is applied directly to the wound with a Q-tip applicator. Hemostasis is achieved in a matter of seconds for superficial oozing. Monsel's solution (20% ferric subsulfate) may be used, but iron deposition can cause tattooing of the skin. For more profuse bleeding, gentle electrocautery should be used, although it can result in a greater risk of scarring.

8. The biopsy site is cleaned with hydrogen peroxide or tap water and petrolatum or an antibiotic ointment is placed under a Band-Aid.

9. Wound-care instructions consist of cleaning the site once a day with tap water followed by the application of an ointment such

TABLE 5-3

Instructions for Wound Care After a Skin Biopsy
1. Remove the Band-Aid after 24 hours.
2. Cleanse the biopsy site daily with soap and water. Pat dry. Then apply a small dab of ointment (e.g., Polysporin) and cover with a new Band-Aid.
3. It is important not to let a scab form. *Do not* leave the wound open to the air! This will delay healing.
4. Continue wound care until healed, approximately 5–7 days.
5. If you have any problems, please call _____.
6. Comments _____
Source: Courtesy of the Yale Dermatologic Surgery Unit.

➡ A simple razor blade, split in half and sterilized is an excellent biopsy device. The curvature can be adjusted to match the surface being biopsied.

as Polysporin. The patient should be instructed to continue wound care until the area has completely healed over with new skin. A uniform pink or red wound is usually seen as soon as epithelialization is complete. Many patients still believe that a wound should be exposed to the air and a scab should be allowed to form. Patients should be educated that moist occlusion will allow quicker healing of the wound. Table 5-3 is a sample wound-care instruction sheet.

CURETTE BIOPSY

The curette is an infrequently used method of skin biopsy. Its major advantage is ease and rapidity. The efficacy of the curette results from its ability to easily separate pathologic tissue from normal skin. The curette is used for superficial lesions only and is most useful for exophytic growths such as warts, keratoses, and skin cancers. Curettage does not interfere with subsequent treatments. The major disadvantage of curettage as a biopsy technique is that insufficient tissue may be obtained. Depth of invasion and margins are impossible for the pathologist to accurately assess. A potential advantage using the curette is that it may provide definitive treatment of the lesion.

Curettes are available in various sizes and shapes. The curette has a semisharp cutting edge that easily cuts through friable tissue but is not sharp enough to cut into the normal dermis. The curette thus allows superficial growths to "shell out" by separating the softer skin growth from underlying firm dermis. Curettage results in minimal destruction to normal tissue and often produces the least apparent scar.

To use the curette correctly takes some practice. Experience will help you to appreciate its "feel." The curette should be held firmly and pressed aggressively across the lesion. It should rest in your hand as would a pencil. A common mistake is not to be firm enough with its movement and use. The curette should be drawn in a steady and firm manner through the lesion in a downward scraping and scooping motion that separates the lesion from the underlying normal dermis [Figure 5-4]. Traction should be placed on the surrounding skin with the opposite hand, which helps to create tension on the surface. The curette works best on a firm surface (forehead or nose) and is difficult to use on a soft surface (eyelid or lip). Bleeding is controlled in the usual fashion by the methods outlined in Table 5-2).

The curette is a versatile device that permits biopsies, or removal

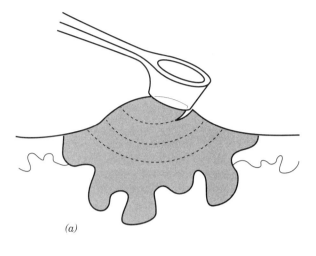

(a)

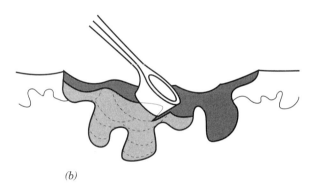

(b)

Figure 5-4. Curette
The curette is an excellent device for the biopsy and removal of superficial lesions. The curette can be either a disposable item, which tends to be the sharpest, or a reusable one. The sharp edge permits the curettage of the skin specimen and may also be used for therapeutic purposes by scraping away the lesion and following with cauterization.

(a) After anesthesia is obtained, gently scrape off the lesion by pulling the curette in a single swift motion.

(b) If the tissue is soft and residual material remains, repeat the process described in (a). In addition, repeat passes will help define the periphery of the lesion.

of superficial lesions in their entirety but your success will depend on experience. It is important to develop a tactile sense of the curette against the skin and be familiar with variation in skin thickness. To perform curettage, proceed as follows:

1. Mark the borders of the lesion with an indelible marker such as a Sharpie fine point pen.

2. Clean the surface with antiseptic if indicated.

3. Inject anesthetic solution directly under lesion to be curetted.

4. Wait several minutes for the vasoconstrictor to become effective.

5. With the curette held like a pencil in your dominant hand, spread the skin and keep it taut using your other hand. Alternatively

an assistant can do this but the vibration from the curette as you feel it in your fingertips helps you gauge the depth of curetting.

6. Pass the curette over the surface of the lesion attempting gently to remove the top surface. Wipe away debris.

7. Repeat the curettage defining the periphery of the lesion.

8. If you are going to combine dessication in the procedure to destroy a malignant lesion, do it gently now.

9. If you have removed a benign lesion for cosmetic reasons, avoid cautery. Apply aluminum chloride. Avoid iron-containing compounds that can tattoo.

10. If the curette penetrates through the skin into the subcutis during treatment of a skin cancer, it is an indication that the tumor is too deep and must be excised.

11. Upon completion of normal curettage, normal dermis should be visible, identifiable by its white color and presence of residual follicles.

SCISSORS BIOPSY

The scissors biopsy is a variant of the shave biopsy and is indicated for superficial, pedunculated, and exophytic skin growths (skin tags, filiform warts, papular keratoses). Local anesthesia may not be necessary if the base of the lesion is small. Forceps with teeth are used to gently grasp and elevate the lesion and sharp iris scissors (curved are preferable) are used to cut the lesion at the base so that it is flush with the surrounding skin [Figure 5-5].

PUNCH BIOPSY

The punch biopsy entails the removal of a cylindrical, full-thickness skin sample utilizing a specialized cutaneous punch trephine (see Chapter 7). A punch biopsy may be incisional or excisional depending on the lesion's size and the size of the punch. A punch biopsy is quick, although the occasional need for sutures requires more time than a simple shave biopsy. Advantages of a punch biopsy include a full-thickness (epidermis to fat) specimen, quick healing,

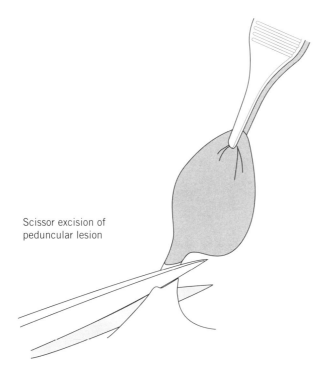

Figure 5-5. Scissors Excision
Scissors excision can be performed as demonstrated and permits the rapid removal of many superficial lesions.

and good cosmesis (with suture repair). Disadvantages include limited size and limitation of depth.

The punch biopsy can only go as deep as the length of the cylinder and is therefore inadequate to sample deeper fat or fascia. Larger-diameter punches (5 mm and 6 mm) will result in dog-ear deformities when the defect is closed with sutures unless steps are taken at the time of the biopsy to convert the circular defect into an ellipse by applying perpendicular tissue traction.

The punch biopsy is commonly used for diagnosis of inflammatory skin diseases and certain neoplastic conditions. It is the biopsy of choice when diagnosing an invasive squamous cell carcinoma or morpheaform basal cell carcinoma. If more than a superficial specimen is required, a punch biopsy should always be performed. A punch biopsy can also be helpful to provide specimens for tissue culture, immunofluorescence, and electron microscopy. Special transport media are required for these more specialized biopsies.

The technique for a punch biopsy is as follows [Figure 5-6]:

1. The site may be prepared with 70% isopropyl alcohol, Betadine, or chlorhexidine.

Skin Biopsy

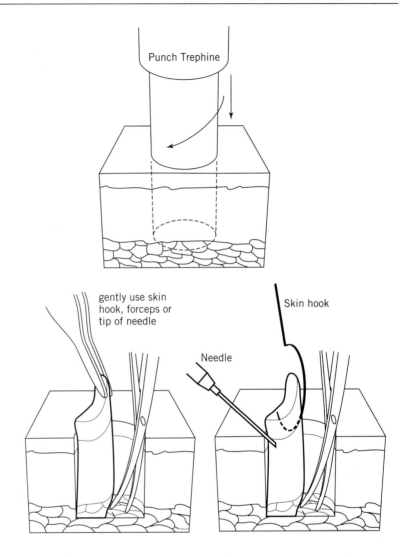

Figure 5-6. Punch Biopsy
Punch biopsy permits standardized removal of a specific amount of tissue involving the epidermis, dermis, and deeper tissues. A skin hook or forceps may be used to immobilize punch specimen for elevation and removal.

2. Local anesthesia is performed in a typical manner utilizing 1% or 2% lidocaine. Epinephrine added to the lidocaine (see section on Anesthesia) is very helpful to limit bleeding and helps visualization during specimen removal.

3. Punch biopsy instruments come in a variety of sizes, ranging from 1.5 mm to 10 mm. The smaller punches (1.5 mm and 2 mm) are excellent on the face where cosmesis is very important. The most commonly used sizes elsewhere are probably 3 mm and 4 mm punches. Punch biopsy instruments are disposable or reusable. The advantage of the disposable punch is consistent sharpness. Reusable

punches dull easily and require frequent sharpening and do not provide any advantages over reusable punches for routine biopsy. The selection of punch size depends on several factors, including the size of the lesion, desire for incisional or excisional biopsy, anatomic location, and preoperative diagnosis.

4. After selecting the appropriate size, the punch is placed perpendicular to the lesion and rotated between the fingers in a circular motion while applying gentle downward pressure. This circular motion can be back and forth in a clockwise and counterclockwise fashion or it can be unidirectional. As the punch descends through dermis into the fat, there is a noticeable decrease in tissue resistance ("give").

5. It is important to place traction on the skin with the opposite thumb and index finger. Lateral tension is placed on the skin perpendicular to the desired long axis of closure. After the punch is taken and the tension is released, the elastic nature of the skin will turn the circular defect into an oval, as illustrated in Figure 5-7. With proper planning, the closure can be properly aligned with relaxed skin tension lines. It is this application of tension that will help minimize dog ears with larger punch biopsies.

6. To avoid histologic artifacts, the cylindrical tissue sample must be removed gently. Plugs of tissue can be atraumatically elevated with forceps, a single-prong skin hook, or a needle such as that used for the local anesthesia. The specimen should be transsected at its deepest base portion with fine-curved iris scissors. Scissors with serrated edges work especially well.

7. The resulting defect will heal by itself, but the best cosmetic results and most rapid healing obtain when the biopsy site is sutured.

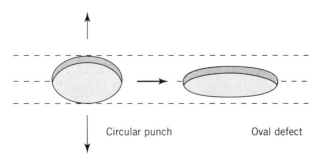

Figure 5-7. Oval Wound
A punch biopsy can be manipulated to create an oval wound so that it will heal without a noticeable circular scar. This is done by providing traction exactly perpendicular to the final axis that is desired.

Simple interrupted or vertical mattress sutures work well. A 2 mm punch will typically require one suture; a 4 mm punch will require two sutures for closure. The sutures are left in place for approximately 4–7 days. They can be removed when the patient returns to the office to check healing of the biopsy site and to discuss the biopsy results. If returning to the office is difficult for the patient, rapidly absorbing 5-0 chromic sutures can be used. These will typically dissolve in 5–7 days. Steri-strips are placed over the biopsy site where the chromic sutures have been placed. The patient is instructed to remove the Steri-strips in 7 days and the residual suture material will be removed as well.

8. Some physicians will allow the punch biopsy site to heal by granulation (second intention). In this case, bleeding needs to be controlled. Gelfoam can be placed directly into the defect for this purpose.

9. A dressing is placed and wound-care instructions are given. The biopsy site should be cleaned on a daily basis with tap water and soap (hydrogen peroxide is toxic to cells in vitro!) and a small amount of antibiotic ointment is placed over the site. Polysporin is preferable to Neosporin as neomycin carries a higher risk of allergic reaction. If the punch biopsy site is in an area of tension, the patient should be instructed to minimize activity to avoid bleeding or wound dehiscence.

EXCISIONAL BIOPSY TECHNIQUE

The technique employed for excisional biopsy is that of conventional elliptical excision. This approach is indicated when a large specimen must be sampled, or if you anticipate that this procedure is both diagnostic and therapeutic. A most important factor to consider when doing an elliptical biopsy is whether your goal is complete removal of the lesion or partial sampling. Once you have identified and marked the lesion, proceed to perform an elliptical excision as described in Chapter 10. Be aware that certain tissue such as the sebaceous skin of the nose, and skin that is disposed to high tension, may best be sampled in ways other than complete fusiform excision. It is important to remember than an "elliptical" biopsy is a bonafide excision and all principles apply.

SPECIAL CONSIDERATIONS

Biopsy of a Suspected Melanoma

If a pigmented lesion is clinically atypical or the differential diagnosis includes melanoma, the lesion should be excised and removed in its entirety with an elliptical excision. A conservative margin (2–3 mm) should be taken and dissection carried down to the subcutaneous tissue. This provides the pathologist with a complete specimen to study for evidence of invasive melanoma. If a melanoma is diagnosed, a full-thickness excision will allow an accurate measurement of the depth of invasion (Breslow depth). The Breslow depth is critical for prognosis, treatment recommendations, and subsequent follow-up regimen. A suspicious pigmented lesion should *not* be removed with a shave biopsy unless the operator is very skilled and can be certain to obtain the full depth of the lesion. In addition, benign pigmented lesions that recur after previous incomplete shave removal may show atypical histologic changes that can be difficult to distinguish from a true melanoma (pseudomelanoma).

For larger pigmented lesions that are difficult to surgically remove (e.g., a 2 cm lentigo maligna on the face), a punch biopsy is indicated. The most atypical-appearing areas should be biopsied (full thickness to fat) or multiple punch biopsies should be taken to minimize potential sampling error. There is no evidence to suggest that incision through a melanoma will increase the risk of metastatic spread of the melanoma.

Oral Biopsy

Biopsies of oral lesions are more challenging because of difficult access in an enclosed space, as well as the risk of bleeding in a highly vascular area. Fortunately, mucosal surfaces heal very well and very quickly. Helpful hints for biopsies of oral lesions include:

1. Use epinephrine and wait 10 minutes to allow for appropriate vasoconstriction and less bleeding.

2. Use a table that tilts back to allow better lighting and easier access.

3. A plastic or metal cheek retractor can be placed over the buccal mucosa to improve access and visualization.

4. A dry 4 × 3 in. gauze to grasp the tongue and/or oral tissue provides improved traction and visibility.

➥ When biopsying a lesion on the mucosa of the lip or cheek, immobilize the lesion with a chalazion clamp. This allows you to manipulate the lesion while minimizing bleeding.

Skin Biopsy

5. A chalazion clamp is very useful for performing biopsies of the distal tongue, lip, or anterior buccal mucosa. The clamp can be gently tightened over the lesion to be biopsied. This provides a firm, movable surface and excellent hemostasis.

6. Due to the tissue vascularity, the biopsy site can be presutured. Silk sutures are usually used for oral biopsies because they lie down flat and are nonirritating. A 5-0 silk suture can first be placed under the lesion into the soft tissue, making sure the needle pass is deep enough. A punch biopsy is then taken and the suture is immediately tied off. This provides for quick hemostasis.

7. The suture should be removed in 5 days as the mucosa heals very rapidly.

Nail Biopsy

Biopsy of the nail is sometimes required to diagnose neoplasms, psoriasis, lichen planus, and mycotic infections. Biopsy of the nail plate, nail bed, nail matrix, nail fold, or hyponychium may be required. Biopsy of the nail matrix may result in permanent nail dystrophy (ridging and splitting) and therefore knowledge of proper technique and anatomy is important. Figure 5-8 shows a cross section of nail anatomy. Nail biopsies should be performed as follows:

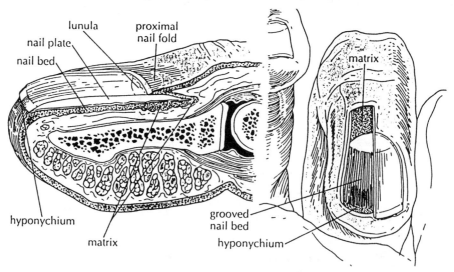

Figure 5-8. Nail Anatomy
The nail consists of the nail plate, nail matrix, nail bed, and nail fold. Reprinted with permission Fewkes J. L., Cheney M. L., and Pollack, S. V, 1992. Illustrated Atlas of Cutaneous Surgery, *Lippincott, Philadelphia.*

1. Before a biopsy is performed, identify and treat any concurrent infection. A firm growth or marked tissue distortion should raise the possibility of a bony abnormality and should prompt an X-ray to look for abnormal bone growths.

2. When possible, obtain the biopsy from the nail bed rather than the nail matrix to avoid potential nail plate deformity.

3. Remove the smallest amount of tissue to make the correct diagnosis. A 3 mm punch is usually adequate in most instances and allows for suture closure and good healing.

4. Local anesthesia is best achieved with a digital block using 2% plain lidocaine.

5. A tourniquet (⅜ in. Penrose drain) can be placed at the base of the finger to control bleeding. Lateral pressure directly over the digital arteries will also control bleeding.

6. A punch biopsy can be performed directly through the nail plate into the nail bed [Figure 5-9]. Pressure or a small piece of Gelfoam will provide hemostasis. However, avulsion of the nail plate permits direct visualization of the nail bed or nail matrix and allows for suture closure.

7. Nail avulsion is the separation of the nail plate from the underlying nail bed and cuticle. This is best accomplished using a dental spatula or nail elevator [Figure 5-10]. After adequate anesthesia is obtained (using a digital block), firm pressure should be applied

➡ A tourniquet is helpful to control bleeding when operating on a finger or toe. A Penrose drain clamped with a hemostat works well, but never leave it in place for more than five minutes, be sure the pressure is not excessive, and never use this technique on a diabetic or other individual with peripheral vascular disease or neuropathy.

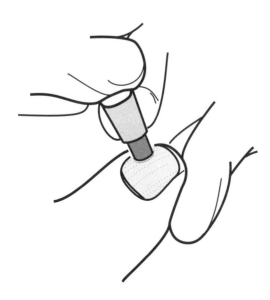

Figure 5-9. Nail Punch
A rapid way to evaluate a pigmented lesion or other suspicious lesions in the nail is to perform a punch directly through the nail plate into the nail bed itself.

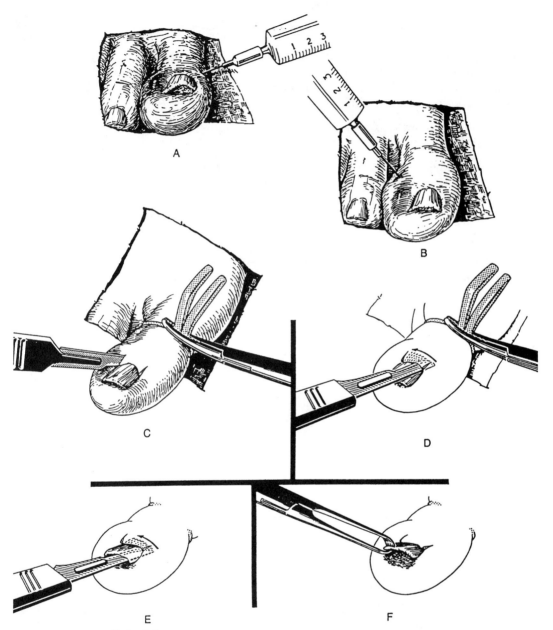

Figure 5-10. Nail Avulsion
After a digital block is obtained, a tourniquet may be placed around the finger for no more than 5 minutes. The nail is loosened from the nail bed with the end of a hemostat, elevator, or scalpel blade. It is then grasped aggressively with the hemostat and twisted in an alternating screwdriver-type fashion while applying withdrawing traction. The nail will then lift and be easily removed. The procedures are remarkably painless with proper anesthesia. Reproduced with permission from Benjamin, R. B., Ed. 1989, Atlas of Office Surgery, *Lea & Febiger, Philadelphia. Illustrations by Alan O. Hage.*

Special Considerations

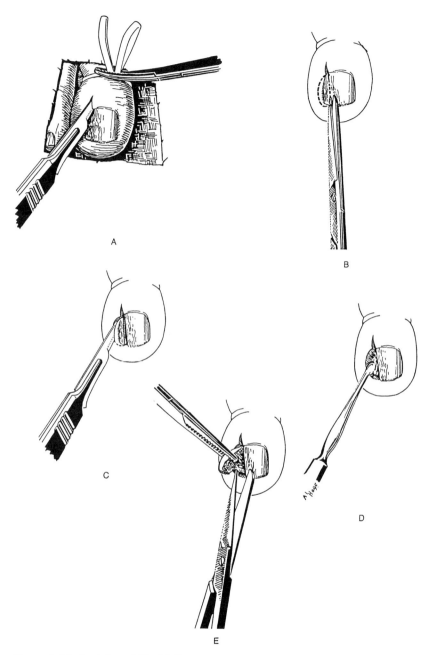

Figure 5-11. Incision of the Nail
Occasionally it is necessary to get an incisional biopsy of the nail bed. In reality it is quite difficult to suture the nail bed and one may, after performing the incision, allow it to heal by second intention. Reproduced with permission from Benjamin, R. B., Ed., 1989, Atlas of Office Surgery, *Lea & Febiger, Philadelphia.*

directly under the distal nail plate to allow the spatula to separate nail plate from nail bed. The instrument should be pushed proximally to the matrix where initial resistance is less. Once over the matrix, the elevator should be pushed gently into the proximal nail groove. Side-to-side longitudinal strokes will free up the nail plate completely. The nail plate is then firmly grasped with a clamp and removed with a back-and-forth rocking motion.

8. For most nail bed lesions, a 3 mm punch is used. The punch should be taken full thickness through the nail bed to the underlying periosteum. Iris scissors are used to free up the specimen. Closure can be performed with interrupted, absorbable sutures.

9. If a larger nail bed specimen is needed, use a longitudinally oriented fusiform excision with a 3 mm width. This will allow for undermining and primary suture closure [Figure 5-11].

10. A nail matrix biopsy may be necessary for nail plate malformations, melanonychia striata, and matrix tumors. When possible, a distal matrix biopsy should be performed because potential deformities will be on the undersurface of the nail plate. A proximal matrix biopsy might result in surface nail plate deformities. A 3 mm punch is typically used and can be closed with absorbable sutures.

11. If a larger fusiform matrix biopsy is required, orient the biopsy transversely in the matrix and avoid the distal lunular edge. Closure can be accomplished with absorbable sutures.

BIOPSY RECORD KEEPING

Once a biopsy is taken, it is important to ensure that both physician and patient receive the results in a timely fashion. It is not adequate to tell the patient to "call back in a week." A system of checks and balances is needed to ensure that the specimen was received at the lab, a report was generated and sent back to the doctor's office, and the results were conveyed to the patient. Documentation is important for obvious medical/legal reasons.

Most offices use a biopsy book or log for keeping track of biopsy specimens and cataloging results. This log should include the patient's name and telephone number, date of the biopsy, location of the biopsy, preoperative diagnosis, type of biopsy performed (shave, punch), which lab the specimen was sent to, special studies requested (e.g., immunofluorescence), final results, date the patient was contacted, and whether further treatment was needed and scheduled.

Use of a simple biopsy card is helpful and becomes part of the permanent chart record. A biopsy card is filled out at the time the biopsy is taken and kept on file by date until the pathology report returns. The pathology report is reviewed by the doctor and the card is appropriately filled out. This method ensures that the report has been reviewed, the patient contacted, and appropriate follow-up arranged.

An occasional problem arises when the patient returns for definitive treatment and the site of the biopsy is difficult to locate. Often it has healed over well or the patient has significant underlying actinic damage that obscures the biopsy site. Skin cancer requiring treatment can persist below the surface even though the biopsy site has healed very well. It is important at the time of the biopsy to carefully mark out on preprinted anatomic sheets where the biopsy was performed. Exact measurements from anatomic landmarks (e.g., 2.5 cm lateral from the alar rim and 3.6 cm inferior to the midpupillary line) are often helpful for locating the biopsy site at a future treatment date. Alternatively, photographic documentation using instant photographic techniques can be very helpful. The Polaroid Spectrum camera with the F112 close-up lens is simple to use and provides photographs of sufficient quality for biopsy site identification.

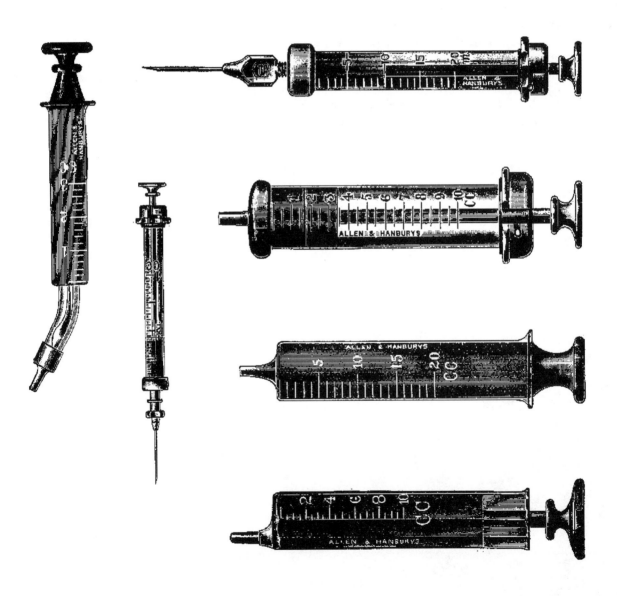

6

Local Anesthesia

In the office setting, the skill of the surgeon is in part measured by the comfort of the patient. Dermatologists have developed many refinements of anesthetic techniques that permit a broad range of office surgical procedures. A thorough understanding of the agents used and the techniques applied will help you achieve the highest measure of comfort for your patient.

Strictly speaking, local anesthesia is the delivery of a pharmacologic agent that causes transient and circumscribed loss of cutaneous sensation without loss of consciousness. Most cutaneous surgery is performed with the aid of local anesthesia.

CHEMISTRY AND CLASSIFICATION

Local anesthetics are divided into two major groups: esters and amides. Both groups have an aromatic portion, an amide portion, and an intermediate chain. The chemical difference between ester and amide anesthetics is the linkage in the intermediate chain. The aromatic portion of a local anesthetic is responsible for lipid solubility, which allows the anesthetic to diffuse through the highly lipophilic nerve membrane. The amide portion is responsible for the hydrophilic properties. Changes in any of these components will change anesthetic potency, onset, and duration of action.

A major difference between amides and esters is their site of metabolism. Esters are hydrolyzed in the plasma by pseudocholines-

Local Anesthesia

terase, whereas amides are degraded in the liver by microsomal oxidases. Patients with hepatic disease may be predisposed to toxicity with amide anesthetics.

A nerve impulse is generated from the movement of sodium and potassium ions across the nerve membrane. Local anesthetics work by preventing sodium channels from opening, thus preventing depolarization and generation of an action potential. Local anesthetics block peripheral nerve function by interfering with the normal excitation and conduction process of nerves.

Table 6-1 lists the ester and amide anesthetics. Lidocaine is by far the most common local anesthetic because of its rapid onset of action and low toxicity. Esters are infrequently used due to their potential for allergic reactions. As a general rule, the longer-acting anesthetics have lower maximal safe dosages as well as a slower onset of action.

Lidocaine comes in multiuse vials with concentrations of 0.5%, 1%, and 2%. It is commercially prepared plain or with epinephrine, usually in 1:100,000 concentration. For most common skin surgery procedures, 1% lidocaine is used; 2% is very useful for nerve blocks. Approximate maximum safe dosages for 1% lidocaine are 30 cc (plain) or 50 cc (with epinephrine). Bupivacaine and etidocaine are longer-acting anesthetics but have a longer onset of action. They are sometimes mixed with lidocaine in an attempt to take advantage of the useful properties of each drug, although mixtures are unpredictable and putative advantages are only theoretical. Mixtures of anesthetic drugs may take on the exclusive properties of only one of the drugs.

> In patients who are considered allergic to lidocaine (a very rare occurrence in reality), inject bacteriostatic saline instead. The perservative has anesthetic qualities and the effect lasts just long enough to do the biopsy.

TABLE 6-1 Common Local Anesthetics

Generic Name	Proprietary Name	Onset	Duration*
Ester Class (plasma metabolism)			
Cocaine		rapid	45
Procaine	Novocain	rapid	15–45
Tetracaine	Pontocaine	slow	120–140
Amide Class (liver metabolism)			
Lidocaine	Xyocaine	rapid	30–120
Mepivacaine	Carbocaine	slow	30–120
Prilocaine	Citanest	slow	30–120
Bupivacaine	Marcaine/Sensorcaine	slow	20–140
Etidocaine	Duranest	rapid	200

* In minutes.

LOCAL ADDITIVES

Vasoconstrictors are added to decrease bleeding, decrease the absorption of anesthetic, lessen toxicity, and increase duration of action. Epinephrine is the most commonly used vasoconstrictor and is usually available commercially at a concentration of 1:100,000. Higher concentrations of epinephrine are associated with increased adverse effects including restlessness, anxiety, tachycardia, palpitations, and increased blood pressure. Advantages and disadvantages of using epinephrine are listed in Table 6-2. Epinephrine should be used cautiously in patients with underlying cardiac disease and a concentration of 1:200,000 or less should be used. Phenylephrine (pure alpha-agonist) can be used instead of epinephrine for patients with clinically important underlying cardiac disease.

The full vasoconstrictive effects of epinephrine tend to occur after 7–15 minutes. Although the onset of action of lidocaine is very rapid, one should wait an average of 10 minutes to obtain the vasoconstrictor effects of epinephrine. Local ischemia and necrosis have been described with epinephrine but almost always involve the digits. Therefore, vasoconstrictors should *not* be used on the fingers or toes. Epinephrine should also be avoided on the glans penis. Contrary to some commonly held beliefs, it is safe to use epinephrine on the nasal tip and ear. Vasoconstrictors should be used cautiously for large flap and graft procedures because of their effect on vascularity.

Acidic preservatives are added to commercially prepared anesthetic solutions to prevent epinephrine degradation, but acidic solutions can cause more pain with injection. Epinephrine can be mixed fresh each day. To decrease pain on injection, ampules of 1:1,000 epinephrine can be used to make a solution with a higher pH. Although the solution will not have any appreciable shelf life, there

TABLE 6-2 Epinephrine

Advantages	Disadvantages
Decrease bleeding	Delayed bleeding
Decrease absorption	Increased blood pressure
Prolong duration	Palpitations; tachycardia
Lessen toxicity	Anxiety, restlessness
	Aggravate underlying cardiac disease

➥ The pain of anesthesia can be minimized by buffering the lidocaine solution with sodium bicarbonate. In addition, if the solution is warmed to 37°C, the pain of injection is lessened.

will be less pain on injection because it is more alkaline. A total of 0.2 cc (1 : 1,000 epinephrine) is added to a bottle of 20 cc plain lidocaine to give a final concentration of 1 : 100,000. If a concentration of 1 : 200,000 is desired, then 0.1 cc (1 : 1,000 epinephrine) is added to a 20 cc bottle. *A potential hazard of this method is that incorrect amounts of epinephrine may be added.* Only well-trained medical personnel should prepare the customized solutions and all anesthetic bottles must be clearly marked and labeled. Freshly prepared epinephrine solutions should be discarded at the end of the day.

The pain of lidocaine injections can also be minimized by adding sodium bicarbonate to the commercially prepared solution. The acidic pH of a lidocaine and epinephrine solution can be partly neutralized by adding 1 cc of an 8.4% sodium bicarbonate stock solution for every 10 cc of lidocaine solution. Due to the more rapid degradation of epinephrine in this neutralized solution, it should be discarded after 1 week.

ALLERGIC REACTIONS

It is not uncommon for patients to state that they have an allergy to Novocain. Unfortunately, the term *Novocain* has become a generic equivalent for local anesthetics, despite its infrequent use today. Allergic reactions to the esters (Novocain) are well described and are felt due to the metabolite, para-amino benzoic acid (PABA), a common sensitizing agent. True allergic reactions to the amide group (e.g., lidocaine) are quite rare. Less than 1% of all reactions are truly allergic in nature and may be due to added preservatives, especially parabens. Allergic reactions attributed to the amides may actually be reactions to the epinephrine (palpitations, lightheadedness) and/or a vasovagal response to the injection itself. There is no cross reactivity between the amides and ester groups.

If a true allergy to lidocaine is suspected, antihistamines or saline can be used for smaller procedures. Diphenhydramine in a concentration of 12.5 mg/cc can be used intradermally. Onset of anesthesia is rapid, but of short duration. Some cases of tissue necrosis have been reported with this method. Because of potential drowsiness, the patient should not drive after the procedure.

ADVERSE EFFECTS AND DRUG INTERACTIONS

Toxicity of local anesthetics is directly related to the plasma concentration of each drug. Toxic drug levels usually result from the injection of excessive amounts of anesthetic, injection into a highly vascular area (e.g., the scalp), or direct and inadvertent injection into a vessel. For plain lidocaine, the maximum safe dosage is 3–5 mg/kg; with epinephrine, 5–7 mg/kg. For children, 1.5–2 mg/kg is recommended for plain lidocaine and 3–4.5 mg/kg for lidocaine with epinephrine.

Toxic reactions to local anesthetics occur primarily in the central nervous system and cardiac system. Subjective symptoms occur at plasma concentrations of 3–5 μg/ml and include tingling, circumoral numbness, metallic taste, lightheadedness, and scotomata. Objective signs occur at concentrations of 6–10 μg/ml and include slurred speech, disorientation, irritability, nystagmus, tremor, and muscle twitching. With increasingly toxic levels, seizures followed by respiratory depression can occur. Diazepam is the drug of choice to treat seizures. See Table 6-3.

Cardiovascular toxicity can occur, but is less common than the central nervous system side effects. Local anesthetics are vasodilators (with the exception of cocaine, which is a vasoconstrictor) and can cause a decrease in blood pressure. The addition of epinephrine, however, usually prevents this side effect. Cardiac conduction can rarely be affected.

TABLE 6-3 Lidocaine Toxicity

Signs and Symptoms	Concentration
Lightheadedness Circumoral numbness; tingling Scotomata Restlessness	3–6 μg/ml
Nausea, vomiting Tremors Blurred vision Tinnitus Confusion	5–9 μg/ml
Seizures	8–12 μg/ml
Respiratory arrest Coma	12–20 μg/ml

To prevent toxic reactions, it is important to limit the total dose of anesthetic and to be aware of safe maximum concentrations. Lidocaine should be injected slowly and carefully, especially in vascular areas, and a vasoconstrictor should be added to decrease the rate of absorption of the drug.

Vasovagal reactions are diagnosed by the occurrence of sweating, lightheadedness, pale complexion, or nausea. Immediately place the patient in the Trendelbenburg position and place a cold cloth on the forehead. Obtain vital signs as a baseline and engage the patient in conversation. Offer a glass of cold water. The vagal patient will invariably partake.

Tricyclic antidepressants enhance the effects of epinephrine by blocking the reuptake of norepinephrine at nerve endings. This can result in possible increases in blood pressure and pulse rate. Propranolol (a beta-blocker) and lidocaine may rarely conspire to cause a hypertensive reaction followed by reflex bradycardia. This is an idiosyncratic drug reaction and cannot be predicted.

LOCAL ANESTHESIA TECHNIQUE

The basic goal of local anesthesia is to numb the skin and soft tissue in the safest and least painful way. Helpful approaches include the following:

1. *Use a 30 gauge needle.* This small-calibre needle should be used routinely for cutaneous surgery. Although mostly used by dermatologists, it is routinely available from supply houses in ½ in. and 1 in. lengths. Better control is achieved with the ½ in. needle, but larger areas can be more easily anesthetized with the 1 in. needle.

2. *Inject slowly.* There is no doubt that slow injection of the anesthetic agent hurts less. This is probably the single most important way to minimize the pain of injection. Warming the solution to 37°C–41°C is also reported to decrease the pain of injection.

3. *Deeper injections into the subcutis hurt less than intradermal injections.* However, injections in the subcutaneous tissue do take longer to achieve anesthesia, so one must usually wait 10–15 minutes for peak effect. Intradermal injections are more rapid but they also distort local tissue and can be more painful.

4. If possible, *introduce the needle tip through a dilated pore.* This

➥ On sebaceous skin, the pain of anesthetic injection can be minimized by placing the needle directly into a pore.

is helpful when working on sebaceous skin such as the nose. This will minimize the pain associated with the needle stick.

5. *Use the smallest amount of anesthetic possible.* This will minimize tissue distortion of the surgical area and minimize toxicity.

6. *Smaller syringes make slower injections easier to perform.* Use a Luer-lok syringe to assure that the needle stays in place. Best control is often achieved with a 1 or 3 cc syringe.

7. *Topical anesthetics such as EMLA (Eutectic Mixture of Local Anesthetic) sometimes minimize the pain of the needle stick.* Ice cube application is especially helpful in children. Keep the ice cube in place on the skin while the needle is inserted beneath it.

8. *Minimize the total number of needle punctures* by infiltrating a large area and moving the needle in a fan shape [Figure 6-1]. When reinserting the needle, try to do so into an area that has already been numbed.

9. When working in a vascular area or near a known vessel, *pull back on the syringe after insertion* to guard against inadvertent vascular entry and injection.

10. *Talk to the patient during needle insertion and injection.* This helps to allay anxiety.

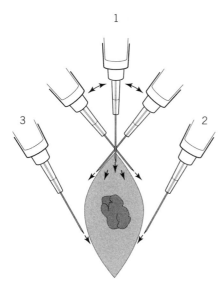

Figure 6-1. Fan Distribution
Local anesthetic is invariably uncomfortable for patients despite all attempts at minimizing it. Use of the fan distribution prevents multiple sticks of the needle, which are actually most painful to the patient. By advancing the needle into a broad area and then withdrawing it partially and reintroducing it in a fanning motion, pain can be minimized.

Local Anesthesia

▶ When anesthetizing the sole, it hurts less if you inject through the dorsal surface.

11. *Squeezing or pinching the area to be injected* will sometimes minimize the pain of the needle stick by providing a counterirritant.

12. *Use fresh epinephrine and/or a bicarbonate solution* to minimize the pain of injection.

13. *If longer procedures are anticipated, use bupivacaine or etidocaine* after first using lidocaine to produce anesthesia.

14. *For extremely anxious patients, consider using anxiolytic drugs* (e.g., Valium) to relieve the anxiety. This can be given sublingually and the effect is obtained within minutes.

Ring Block

A ring block is useful when direct needle entry into a lesion such as a cyst is not desirable. The anesthetic is infiltrated peripherally around the lesion and achieves effective anesthesia, even though no drug was injected into the central area [Figure 6-2]. Such a field block can minimize the total amount of anesthetic used and also minimize tissue distortion.

Nerve Block

Peripheral nerve block involves the injection of a small amount of anesthetic around the nerve to produce anesthesia in the distribution of that nerve. In cutaneous surgery, peripheral nerve blocks are commonly used to anesthetize the fingers, toes, and regions served by the trigeminal nerve of the face. The advantages of a nerve block include numbing large areas with a small amount of drug and minimizing pain, drug toxicity, and tissue distortion. Disadvantages

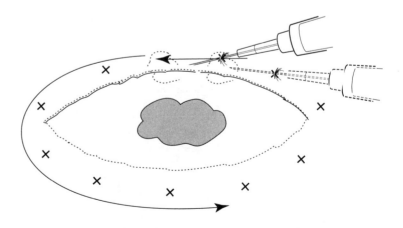

Figure 6-2. Ring Block
The ring block is performed by anesthetizing the periphery of the lesion without direct injection into or under the lesion.

include longer onset time, lack of a vasoconstrictive effect, and risk of direct nerve injury. For nerve blocks 2% lidocaine is typically used.

Needle injection on the fingertips and toes is very painful. Two to three cc of 2% lidocaine (without epinephrine) injected at the base of the finger will successfully anesthetize the entire finger. Each digit is supplied by two superior and inferior digital nerves located laterally and medially. The 30 gauge needle enters at the dorsal lateral aspect of the digit and anesthetic is injected in a dorsal and ventral direction [Figure 6-3]. Large volumes of anesthetic (greater than 5 cc) should be avoided due to a possible compression effect in this closed space. The digital artery runs parallel to the digital nerve, so care must be taken to avoid this vessel.

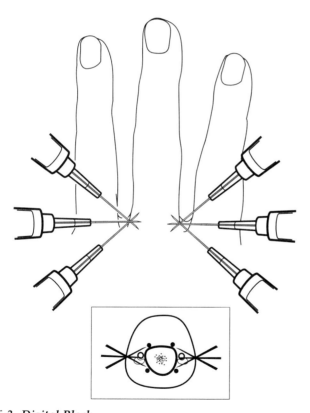

Figure 6-3. Digital Block
Digital block is performed by anesthetizing the digital nerves within the web space. The needle enters the web space at a superior angle. Withdraw from the syringe to make sure that the needle is not in the vessel and infiltrate approximately 1 cc of anesthesia.

A tourniquet can be used at the base of the finger to control bleeding, but it should not be used in diabetics or others with compromised peripheral nerve function. Do not place the tourniquet too tightly or nerve palsy can result. Note the time when the tourniquet was placed and when it must be removed. Epinephrine should not be used.

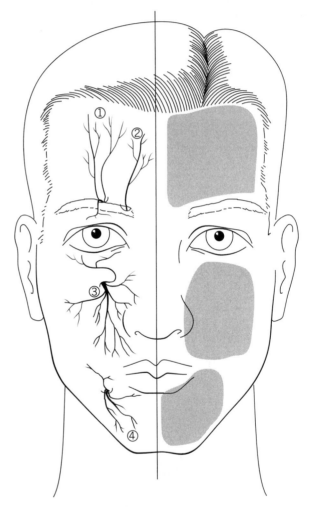

Figure 6-4. Trigeminal Nerve Block
Local installation of anesthetic in these areas can achieve anesthesia over a broad area.

Nerve:	①Supraorbital	②Supratrochlear	③Infraorbital	④Mental
Area supplied:	forehead, upper eyelids	forehead	medial cheek, upper lip, nose, lower eyelids	chin, lower lip

Large areas of the face can be anesthetized using nerve blocks of branches of the trigeminal nerve. Figure 6-4 indicates the location of the supraorbital, supratrochlear, infraorbital, and mental nerves. Note that these nerves are generally located in the midpupillary line.

FOREHEAD. The supraorbital nerve is blocked by injecting 1 cc–2 cc of 2% lidocaine toward (but not in) the supraorbital notch, which lies along the supraorbital ridge in the midpupillary line. The supratrochlear nerve lies at the junction of the nasal root and the upper orbital rim. Nerve block to the supraorbital and supratrochlear nerves will anesthetize the medial forehead from the eyebrow to the scalp.

CHEEK, EYELID, AND NOSE. The infraorbital nerve that supplies sensation to the lower eyelid, medial cheek, nasal side wall, and upper lip exits the infraorbital foramen approximately 1 cm below the infraorbital ridge in the midpupillary line. The foramen is usually palpated without difficulty. Two cc of 1 cc–2% lidocaine is injected around the foramen to achieve anesthesia. The infraorbital nerve can also be approached intraorally in the superior labial sulcus.

CHIN. The mental nerve block will anesthetize the chin and lower lip. The mental nerve exits the mental foramen approximately 2.5 cc from the midline of the face in the midpupillary line. The mental nerve can be blocked on the cutaneous surface or intraorally in the inferior labial sulcus at the apex of the first bicuspid.

TOPICAL ANESTHESIA

Topical anesthetics can be a useful adjunct but cannot completely supplant infiltrative anesthesia for most excisional cutaneous surgical procedures. The major advantages of topical anesthesia are lack of pain, absence of tissue distortion, and decreased risk of systemic absorption and drug toxicity. Topical anesthetics generally work best on mucosal surfaces because of better absorption and on the skin are best used for superficial treatments (e.g., curettage, shave excision). They can also be used to decrease the pain associated with the initial needle stick. Current topical anesthetics include:

1. *Cryoanesthesia,* which refers to the external application of cold to the skin to produce numbness. Ice and refrigerant sprays are typically used. Ice is particularly helpful in children because it is a

➡ For quick biopsies, especially in children or adults fearful of needles, place an ice cube in a latex glove and hold it directly on the skin for about 30–60 seconds. This will provide enough anesthesia for a small shave biopsy.

familiar material of which they are not afraid. Direct application of ice for 30–60 seconds provides rapid, superficial, and very short-duration anesthesia. Keeping the ice cube on the skin while the needle is inserted works well. Injection of the anesthetic will still be felt, but distractive conversation can minimize the sensation. Refrigerant sprays include ethyl chloride and dichlorotetrafluoroethane. Temporary hardening of the skin is a potential problem.

2. Several *topical lidocaine* preparations are available. The newest is EMLA, which is a combination of 2.5% lidocaine and 2.5% prilocaine. A generous amount of EMLA cream should be applied directly to the surgical site and placed under occlusion approximately 3 hours before the procedure. Although the manufacturer suggests a 1-hour application, we have found optimal results when the cream has been in place, occluded by the bandage provided, for 3 hours. EMLA has been reported to be helpful for superficial curettage, epilation, dermabrasion, harvesting of split-thickness skin grafts, pulsed dye laser surgery, and cryosurgery. EMLA is not good for excisional surgery into the subcutaneous tissue. It is recommended that EMLA not be applied to open wounds. Contact sensitivity to both lidocaine and prilocaine has been reported.

Lidocaine is also commercially available as a 2% and 5% jelly and as a viscous solution. These preparations work best on mucosal surfaces. In an acid mantle cream, 30% lidocaine can be compounded and applied under occlusion 1 hour before superficial procedures.

3. *Benzocaine,* an ester anesthetic, is not used for infiltration due to poor water solubility, but is commercially available over the counter as a 20% aerosol spray or gel. Contact sensitivity is a common problem and represents its major disadvantage.

4. *Cocaine* is used as a 2–4% solution applied with cotton balls. It is used almost exclusively for intranasal surgery.

5. When working near the eye, *ophthalmic anesthetics* can be very helpful. Typical agents are 0.5% *tetracaine* or 5.0% *proparacaine.* Two or three drops will effectively anesthetize the corneal surface for 30–60 minutes.

TUMESCENT ANESTHESIA

This technique, initially pioneered for liposuction surgery (wet technique), allows infiltration of large volumes of dilute lidocaine (0.05–

TABLE 6-4 Tumescent Anesthesia

---
1 liter 0.9% sodium chloride
50 ml 1% lidocaine
1 ml 1:1000 epinephrine
12.5 ml sodium bicarbonate
Final concentration: .05% lidocaine, 1:1,000,000 epinephrine

0.1%). Use of this solution allows large areas to be anesthetized safely with concentrations as high as 35–50 mg/kg. Table 6-4 shows the standard formula for tumescent anesthesia. The anesthetic solution is evenly distributed in the subcutaneous layer with a 25-gauge 3-in. needle. Its role in routine office skin surgery has not been well established.

PREANESTHESIA MEDICATIONS

Analgesics and sedatives, are used to decrease anxiety and minimize the pain of the procedure. Conscious sedation is useful if extensive local anesthesia is required. Oral administration of these agents is safer, but tends to be less effective and has a slower onset of action than the same medications given intravenously. Intravenous infusion provides a rapid onset of action and finer control over the desired level of sedation and analgesia. However, it requires close monitoring for signs of respiratory depression.

Diazepam (Valium) is the preferred agent when oral or sublingual administration is desired. Sublingual administration tends to produce a more rapid effect when compared to the oral route. The usual starting dose of diazepam is 5 or 10 mg administered 60 minutes before surgery. It will produce a mild to moderate calming effect on the patient which will make the procedure less stressful. This dosage may be repeated every 3–4 hours as needed. Diazepam has a high safety margin when used orally and is very well tolerated. Intravenous administration of diazepam offers a more rapid onset of action, more predictable anxiolysis, and produces some anterograde amnesia.

The intravenous route is the preferred method of administration when more intense levels of sedation are desired. The injection solution is 5 mg/ml with an initial starting intravenous dose of 2.5–5 mg. This dose can be repeated every 15–20 minutes until a maximum dose of 20 mg is achieved. Most patients require 5–10 mg to achieve the desired sedative effect. By this route, sedation typically lasts about 45 minutes and some element of muscle relaxation and antiseizure effect is also obtained. Common side effects of intravenous diazepam include lightheadedness, motor incoordination, mental impairment, disorganized thought, and ataxia. When used alone, intravenous diazepam has only a moderate depressive effect on respiration. The intravenous administration can cause pain and phlebitis at the injection site.

Midazolam (Versed) provides more rapid onset of action and a shorter recovery time when compared to diazepam. It is also two times more potent than diazepam and is better absorbed after intramuscular injection. The IM dose is .07–.08 mg/kg. Sedative effects will appear in 15 minutes and peak in 30–60 minutes. This IM dosage rarely has an effect on respiration. Anterograde amnesia typically occurs. Intravenous midazolam is less likely to cause phlebitis and does have a faster onset of action compared to diazepam. It can produce a slight decrease in blood pressure. Sedation will occur in 3–5 minutes and lasts for approximately 30 minutes. If used intravenously, a starting dose of 1 mg should be given over 2 minutes. Most normal adults will require a dose of 1–2.5 mg to produce conscious sedation.

Intravenous sedation requires close patient monitoring for signs of respiratory depression and should be performed only by those persons familiar with the use of these agents. Proper management includes a continuous intravenous infusion, pulse oximeter, EKG, and blood pressure monitoring.

At times, it is helpful to use a potent analgesic before surgery if much discomfort is anticipated. Opioids (meperidine, fentanyl) can be given intramuscularly or intravenously, but do produce nausea, vomiting, hypotension, and respiratory depression and should be used with caution. These agents should only be used if resuscitative equipment and naloxone are readily available.

Meperidine can be given as an intramuscular dose of 50–75 mg. Because it may produce nausea and vomiting, it should be given with promethazine or hydroxyzine in dosages of 25–50 mg. Hydroxyzine and promethazine are antihistamines and have an antiemetic effect. Meperidine at lower dosages will provide analgesia and in higher dosages will produce some degree of sedation and euphoria. Serious adverse effects include respiratory depression, seizures, and hypotension.

Fentanyl is a potent morphine-like analgesic that is less likely to produce nausea and vomiting. The analgesic effect has a rapid onset and has a relatively shorter duration of action. The major adverse effect is respiratory depression, which occurs more rapidly than with other morphine-like drugs. Fentanyl is available in ampules containing 50 μg/ml; a typical intramuscular dose is 50–100 μg. Analgesic effect will begin in 7–8 minutes and last 1–2 hours. Fentanyl has less effect on cardiovascular function than other opiates. It is important to note that the vast majority of office cutaneous surgery does not require intravenous or intramuscular analgesics or sedatives. The use of these drugs should only be undertaken if absolutely indicated, by individuals experienced in their administration.

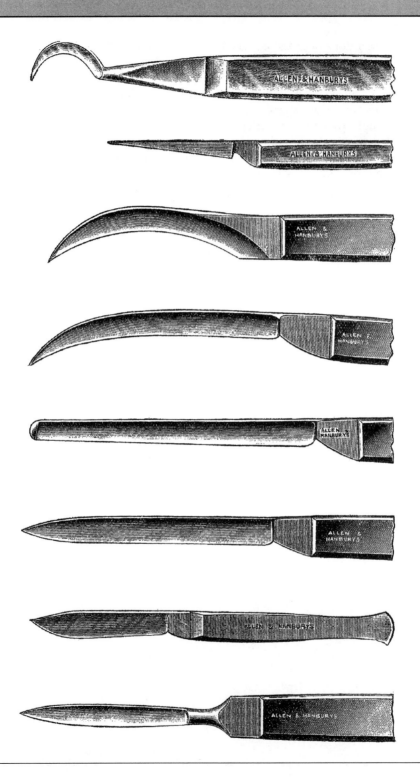

7
Surgical Instruments

It is said that when the only tool you have is a hammer, everything looks like a nail. A well-selected array of surgical instruments will permit you to pursue the correct solution for every problem you encounter. Dermatologic surgical instruments are available in a wide range of quality that varies with the different grades of steel from which they are constructed. Although all instruments are said to be made of stainless steel, this is a misnomer because instruments will rust if not cared for properly. Stainless steel contains carbon alloy, which contributes to hardness, and chromium and nickel are incorporated to help prevent corrosion. The exact concentration of these alloys is adjusted to produce the final product with its characteristics of hardness, corrosion resistance, sharpness, and durability. Some newer materials, such as tungsten carbide, are being incorporated (at increased cost) to enhance durability and function.

As you assemble your surgical instruments, buy quality. Fewer superior instruments are preferable to more of poor quality. Good instruments are expensive. Choose carefully and selectively. Similarly, select a vendor with the highest integrity. It is probably a good idea to request copies of instrument catalogs from a number of sources and compare quality and price. Some well-known companies in the United States include Miltex, Robbins, Tiemann, Storz, VanSickle, Bernsco, and Delasco (see Appendix II). Your surgical instrument is really an extension of your own hand. Similar instruments made by different manufacturers may fit you differently. Go for a test run. Handle a variety of instruments so you can determine which are most comfortable for your surgical tray. [Table 7-1]. As a general rule, instruments for fine cutaneous surgery should be small, lightweight, delicate, and fine tipped.

TABLE 7-1 "Standard" Excisional Surgery Tray

Needle holder
Knife handle (#3)
Blade (#15)
Curette (3 mm)
Iris scissor, curved and straight
Blunt dissecting scissor (e.g., Baby Metzenbaum)
Skin hook (single prong)
Hemostat (mosquito)
Forceps—toothed
Forceps—serrated
Sterile towels
Sterile Q-tips
3 × 4 in. and 2 in. gauze
Sterile basin for Phisoderm or other antiseptic
Hyfrecator cover
Suture material
Towel clamps

SCALPELS

Knife handles and blades are available in a variety of shapes and sizes [Figure 7-1]. The most common knife handle in cutaneous surgery is the flat Number 3 usually used with the Number 15 blade. Knife handles can also be round or octagonal in shape. Some surgeons believe the round handle shape (No. 7) gives better control and comfort as you are able to roll the handle in your fingers without rocking or moving the wrist.

A useful frequent feature of the flat knife handle is a centimeter scale incorporated into the scalpel handle allowing for easy measurement of preoperative and postoperative lesion and wound sizes. The three most common blades are the Number 10, Number 15, and Number 11. The Number 10 blade is a wide blade, curved convexly, which is sharpest on its belly. It is used primarily for larger excisional procedures and permits deep incision, especially on areas like the back where the dermis is particularly thick. The Number 15 blade is the most popular blade and is similar in contour to the Number 10 but is smaller and is sharper at the tip. The Number 15C is a relatively new blade, smaller than the regular Number 15. The Number 11 blade is tapered with a very sharp point and is used mainly

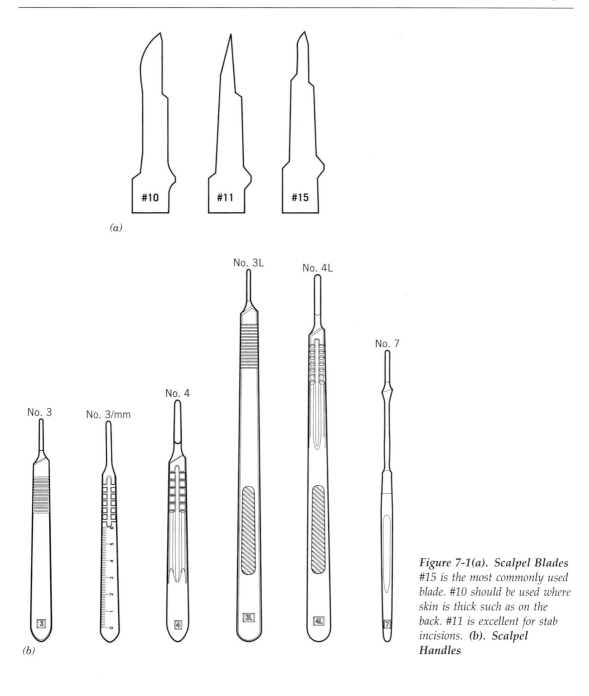

Figure 7-1(a). Scalpel Blades #15 is the most commonly used blade. #10 should be used where skin is thick such as on the back. #11 is excellent for stab incisions. **(b). Scalpel Handles**

for stab incisions (useful in incision and drainage procedures). Disposable handles and blades are also available, but they are not weighted and the blades are usually less sharp.

The Beaver system uses a smaller, narrow, pencil-like handle with a smaller, sharper blade [Figure 7-2]. This handle and blade is excellent for delicate work, especially around the eyes. Its major disadvantage is a more rapid dulling of the blade. The most popular Beaver blade in skin surgery is the Number 67. It is small, convexly curved, and sharp tipped. The Number 64 blade is rounded and has a blunt tip. The Number 65 blade is a smaller version of the Number 11 sharp-point blade.

The Shaw hemostatic scalpel provides hemostasis during cutting of tissue. Standard-size blades are attached to an operator-activated calibrated heat source that heats the scalpel blade and coagulates small blood vessels as it incises tissue. The blades are Teflon coated to prevent sticking.

For personal protection, it is best to remove scalpel blades after use with a blade extractor or hemostat.

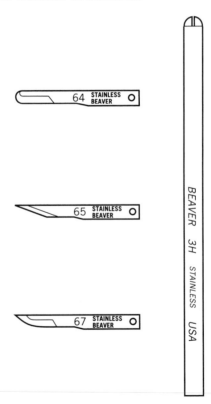

Figure 7-2. Beaver Handle and Blades

NEEDLE HOLDERS

Needle holders come in a variety of sizes and shapes and the nomenclature can be confusing [Figure 7-3]. Many needle holders are eponymous. Comfort and control are essential, especially when doing fine work. In addition, the needle holder is the most abused instrument in the toolbox, due to constant metal-to-metal friction. Needle holders (also called needle drivers) vary in length but most commonly are 4.5–6 inches. The tips and jaws of the needle holder range from wide and blunt to narrow and fine corresponding to needle size and the anatomic area in which the needle and suture is being placed. As a general rule, smaller jaws are used for finer suture material and larger jaws accommodate larger needles and sutures.

The jaws of a needle holder are either smooth or finely serrated. Smooth jaws are considered less damaging to fine-caliber needles. Needle holders can also have cross striations that may permit a more secure grasp of the suture needle. Larger needles can damage the inserts of the small, fine, needle holders and therefore appropriate needle holders should be matched with appropriate needle sizes.

Most skin surgeons prefer to use several sizes of needle holders. One size or type of needle holder will likely not suffice. It is best to use three styles: one for very delicate work, one for regular suturing, and one for tough tissue. Higher-grade (and more costly) instruments have hardened inserts made of tungsten carbide. This alloy is usually indicated by gold handles. The resulting increased strength and hardness of the jaws may provide more secure grasping and less instrument wear. This potential advantage must be weighed against the increased cost. Carbide needle holders are typically guaranteed for 3–5 years.

The Webster and Halsey holders with smooth jaws and tapered tips work very well for small needles and the fine suture material common in skin surgery. The Crile-Wood needle holder has a gently tapered blunt tip and is designed to hold larger needles. Baumgartner and Mayo-Hegar are also used for larger suture needles. A specialized needle holder is the Olsen-Hegar, which has scissors incorporated behind the jaws. This is very convenient when working alone. Be careful not to accidentally cut the suture during the suturing procedure. The Castroviejo needle holder is very useful for areas of delicate suturing such as the periocular region. This needle holder, which has spring handles and an optional self-locking device, is very expensive.

Surgical Instruments

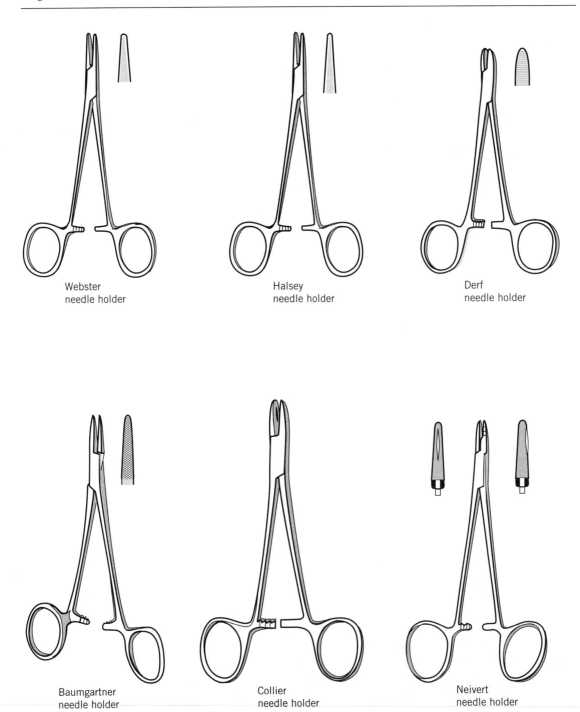

Figure 7-3. Various Needle Holders

FORCEPS

Forceps, also referred to as "pick-ups," are essential in skin surgery. They are used to handle tissue and suture material and are available in a variety of tips for various functions and tissues. Most forceps that you will find helpful are lightweight and fine tipped. They may be either toothed or serrated [Figure 7-4]. Strictly speaking, serrated forceps are referred to as dressing forceps. Although they are excellent for handling gauze and similar materials, their firm grasp of tissue can exert excessive pressure that results in crush injury and potentially significant tissue damage. Toothed forceps commonly have one to three teeth that insert between opposing members to allow gentle grasping of tissue and suture material. One of the more common forceps is the Adson. It has broad handles that taper to a long narrow tip. The Brown-Adson forceps have seven or eight interlocking teeth distributed over the length of the tip to allow for stabilizing thicker tissue.

There are also specialized forceps available. The Bishop-Harmon has three holes in the handle, which make it very lightweight, but this fine-tipped instrument is very delicate and easily bent. Jewelers forceps have a fine, sharp point and are used commonly in hair transplantation surgery. Splinter forceps have superfine, smooth tips and are popular for suture removal. Most forceps can be ordered with tips that are delicate (0.6 mm or less), regular (1–1.5 mm) or heavy (1.6 mm or larger).

SKIN HOOKS

Skin hooks permit atraumatic handling of tissue and are available in varying lengths. The curvature of the tips and degree of sharpness also vary. They can be single, double, or multiple pronged [Figure 7-5]. The multiple-pronged skin hooks are sometimes referred to as "rakes." Skin hooks are extremely useful for manipulating flaps and reflecting wound edges while undermining. They permit easy visualization for hemostasis and placement of deep sutures. The single-pronged, sharp-tipped, skin hook is the most popular among dermatologic surgeons. Common names of skin hooks include Frazier, Tyrrell, Guthrie, and Joseph.

Surgical Instruments

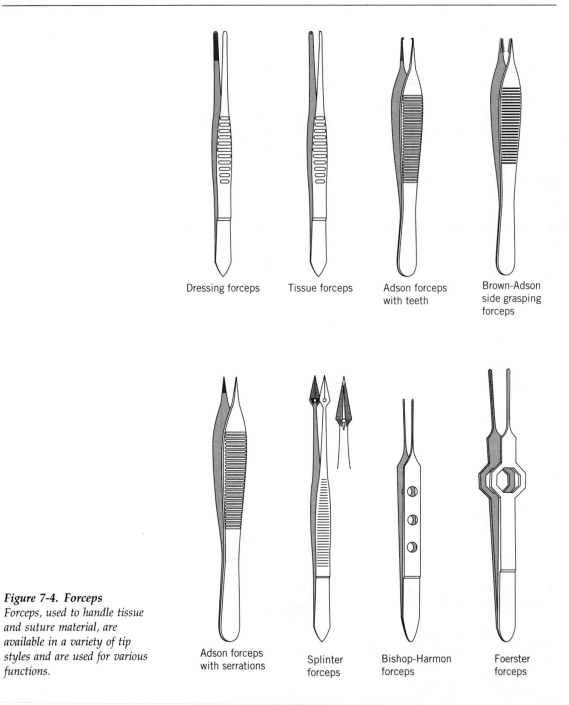

Figure 7-4. Forceps
Forceps, used to handle tissue and suture material, are available in a variety of tip styles and are used for various functions.

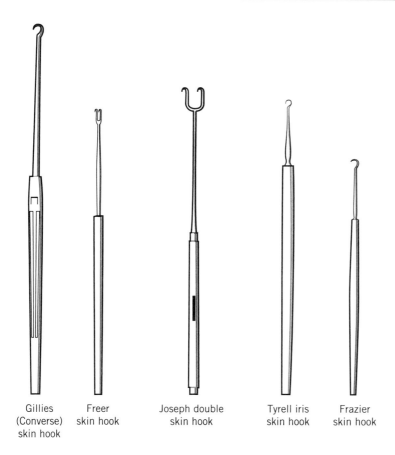

Figure 7-5. Skin Hooks
Examples of skin hooks used for atraumatic handling of tissue.

HEMOSTATS

Hemostats are used to clamp bleeding blood vessels that do not respond to simple electrocoagulation. At times, small arterial bleeders are encountered and the hemostat is essential to identify, grasp, and contain the bleeding. The vessel can then be eletrocoagulated or suture ligated. Hemostats can be straight or curved. For delicate skin surgery, the hemostat should be small, lightweight, and fine tipped. The Halsted hemostat, also referred to as a mosquito hemostat, is an excellent choice [Figure 7-6]. The Hartman and Jacobson work equally well. Hemostats need only be 4 or 5 inches long for cutaneous surgery.

Surgical Instruments

SCISSORS

Scissors come in a vast array of sizes and shapes which can be confusing [Figure 7-7]. Scissors are required in skin surgery for cutting tissue, cutting sutures, undermining tissue, removing sutures, and removing bandages and dressings. Scissors may have long or short handles with blades that are straight or curved. Tips can be blunt (used for undermining) or sharp (used for cutting). The tips can also be smooth or serrated. Serrated tips will cause less

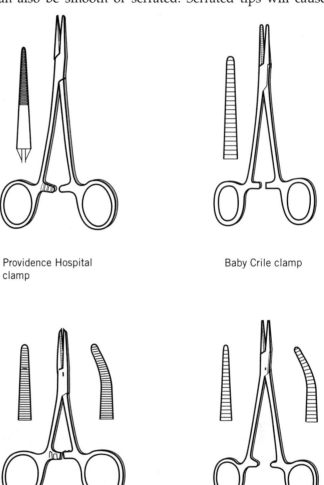

Providence Hospital clamp

Baby Crile clamp

Hartman mosquito clamp

Halsted mosquito clamp

Figure 7-6. Forceps
Examples of hemostatic forceps, or hemostats, used for clamping blood vessels.

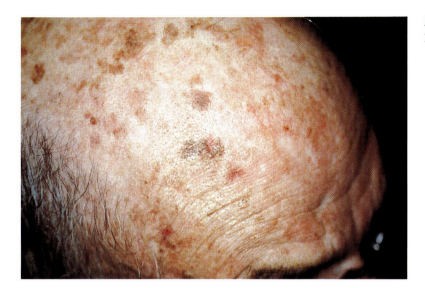

Figure 2-2
Page 9

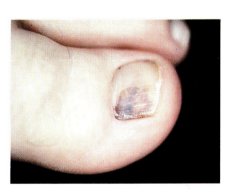

Figure 2-3
Page 10

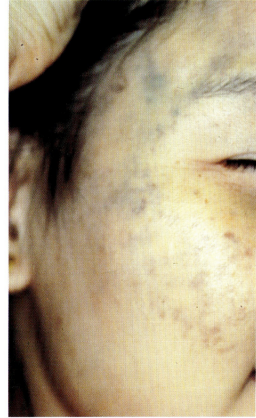

Figure 2-5
Page 11

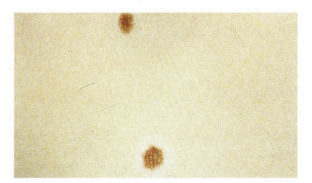

Figure 2-4
Page 10

For complete figure caption, see the page number(s) indicated.

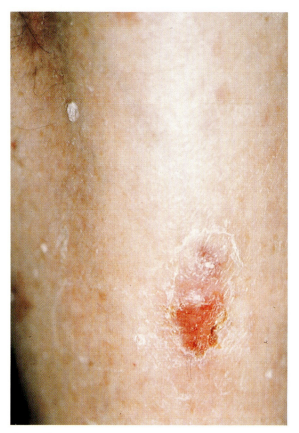

Figure 2-6
Page 11

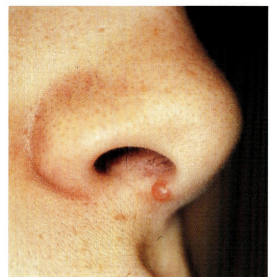

Figure 2-7
Page 12

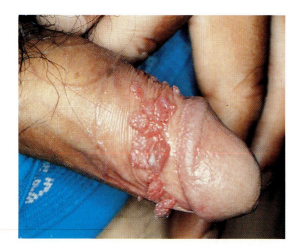

Figure 2-8
Page 12

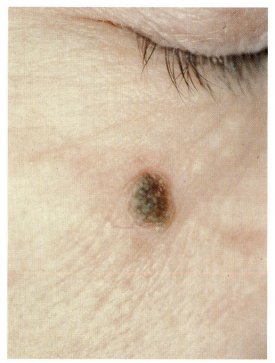

Figure 2-9
Page 13

For complete figure caption, see the page number(s) indicated.

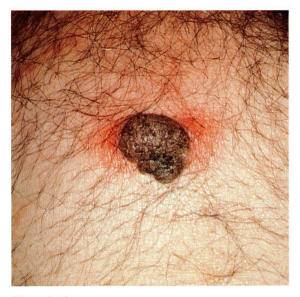

Figure 2-10
Page 14

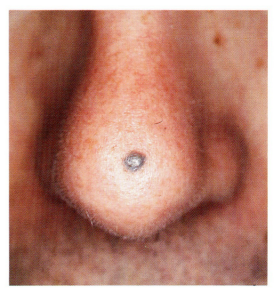

Figure 2-11
Page 14

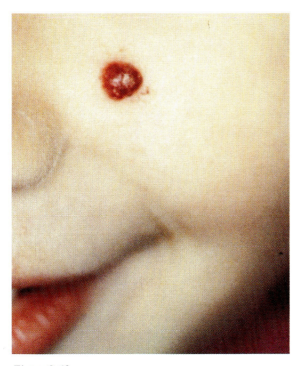

Figure 2-12
Page 15

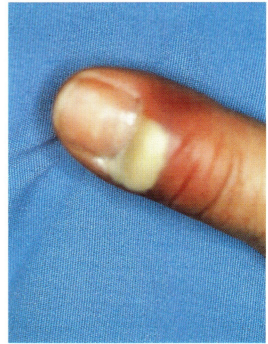

Figure 2-13
Page 16

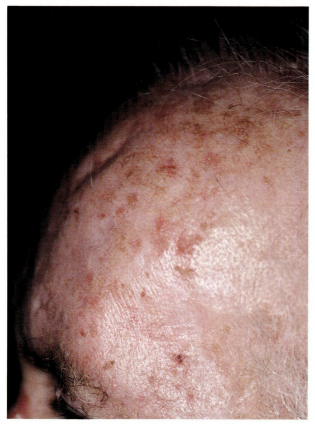

Figure 2-14
Page 17

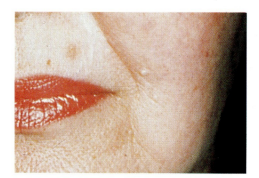

Figure 2-15a
Page 18

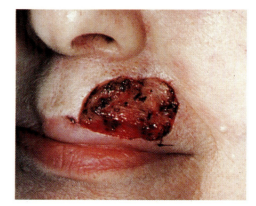

Figure 2-15b
Page 18

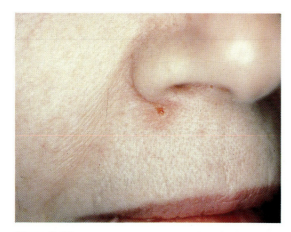

Figure 2-16
Page 19

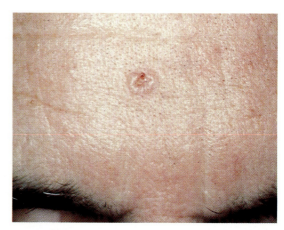

Figure 2-17
Page 19

For complete figure caption, see the page number(s) indicated.

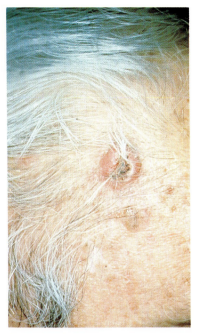

Figure 2-18
Page 20

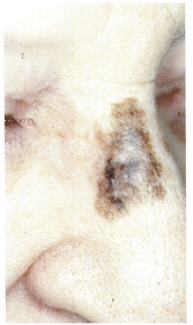

Figure 2-19
Page 21

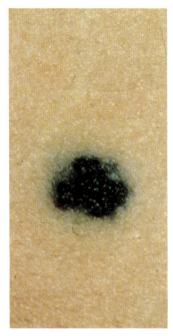

Figure 2-20
Page 22

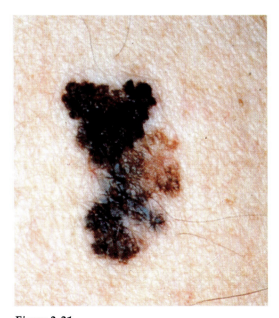

Figure 2-21
Page 22

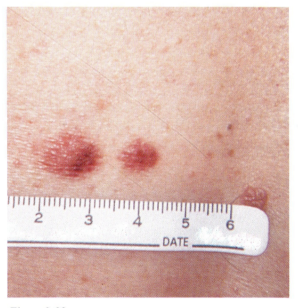

Figure 2-22
Page 23

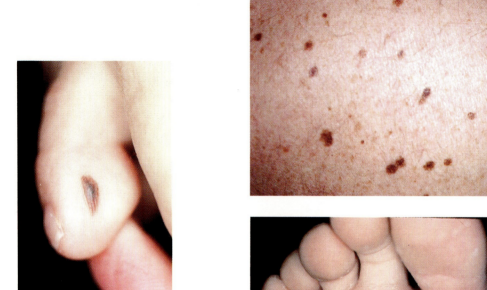

Figure 2-24
Page 25

Figure 2-23
Page 24

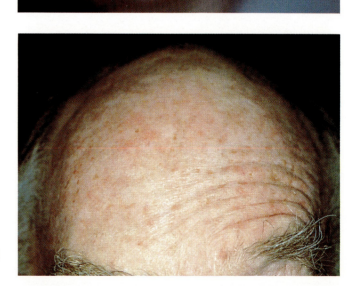

Figure 2-25
Page 28

Figure 3-11
Page 46

For complete figure caption, see the page number(s) indicated.

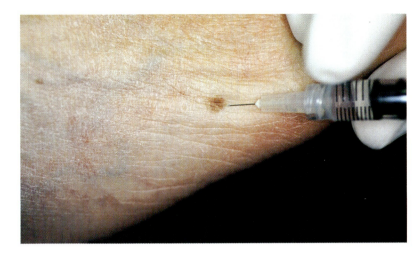

Figure 5a
Page 65

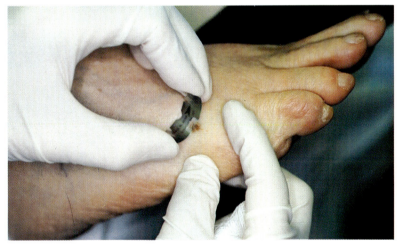

Figure 5b
Page 65

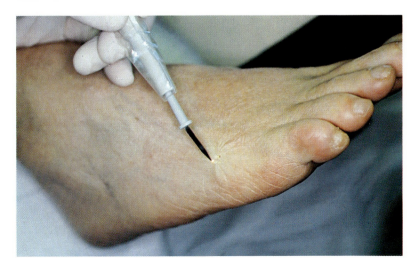

Figure 5c
Page 65

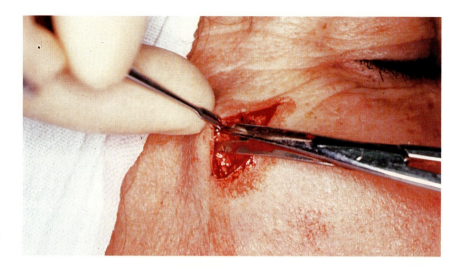

Figure 10-13a
Page 167

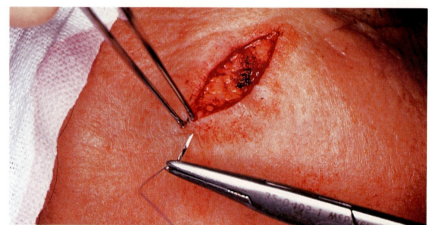

Figure 10-13b
Page 167

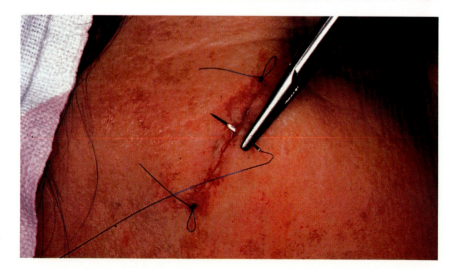

Figure 10-13c
Page 167

For complete figure caption, see the page number(s) indicated.

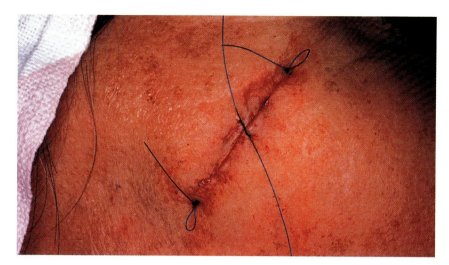

Figure 10-13d
Page 167

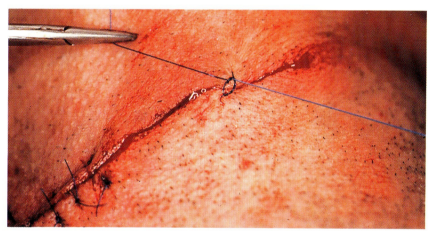

Figure 10-13e
Page 167

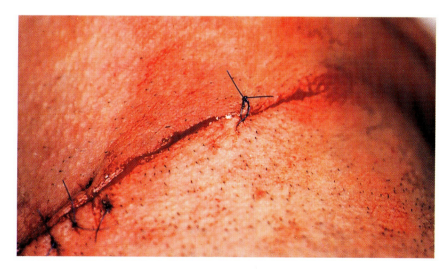

Figure 10-13f
Page 167

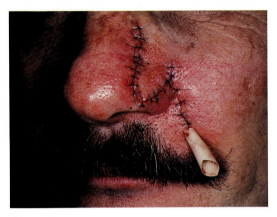

Figure 11-2a
Page 184

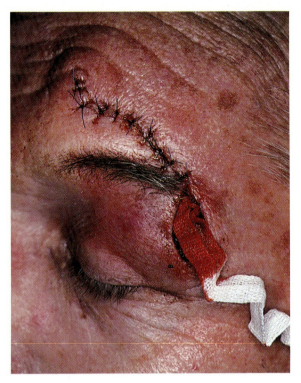

Figure 11-2b
Page 184

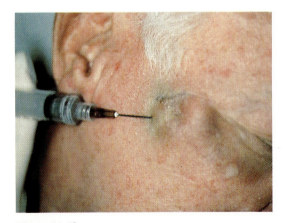

Figure 11-3a
Page 187

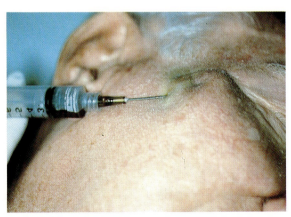

Figure 11-3b
Page 187

Figure 11-3c
Page 187

For complete figure caption, see the page number(s) indicated.

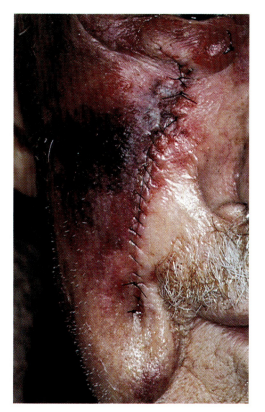

Figure 11-4
Page 188

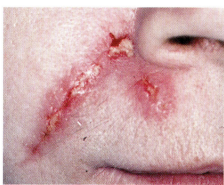

Figure 11-5
Page 190

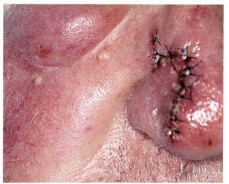

Figure 11-6
Page 190

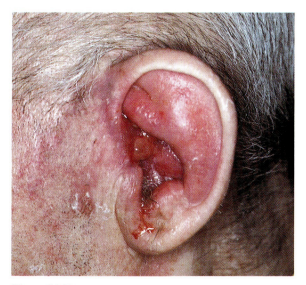

Figure 11-7a
Page 193

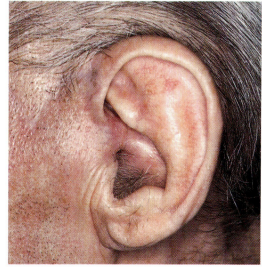

Figure 11-7b
Page 193

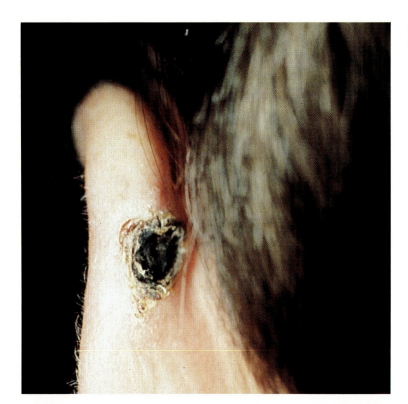

Figure 11-8
Page 195

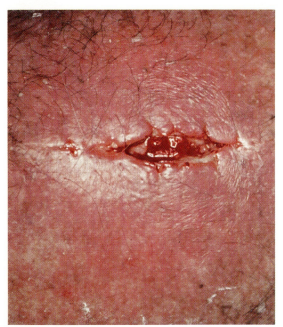

Figure 11-9a
Page 196

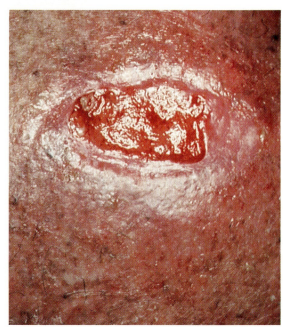

Figure 11-9b
Page 196

For complete figure caption, see the page number(s) indicated.

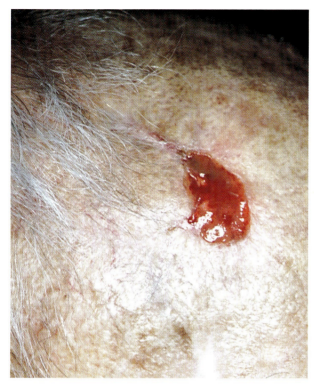

Figure 11-10
Page 198

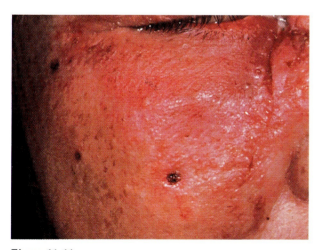

Figure 11-11
Page 199

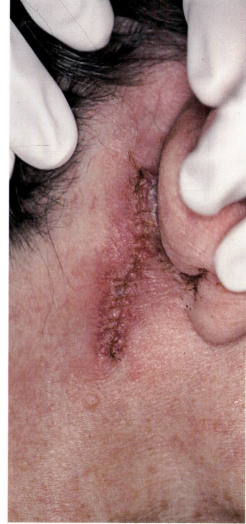

Figure 11-12
Page 202

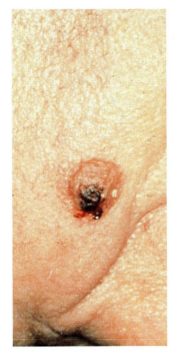

Figure 12-1a
Page 206

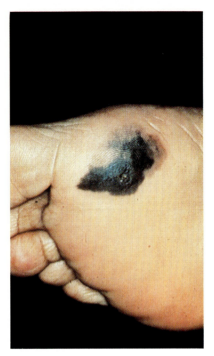

Figure 12-1b
Page 206

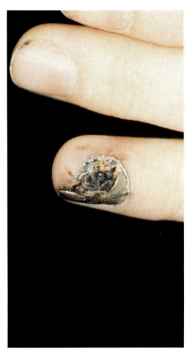

Figure 12-1c
Page 206

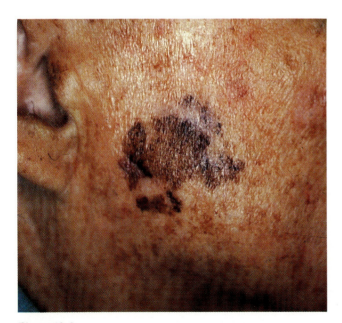

Figure 12-2
Page 210

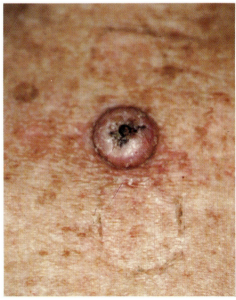

Figure 12-4
Page 214

For complete figure caption, see the page number(s) indicated.

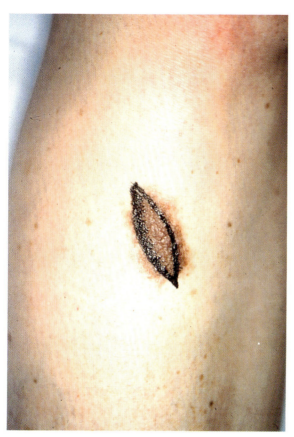

Figure 12-3a
Page 212

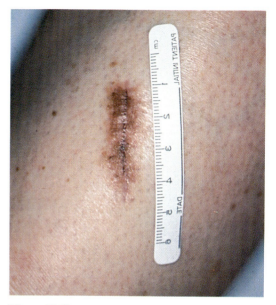

Figure 12-3b
Page 212

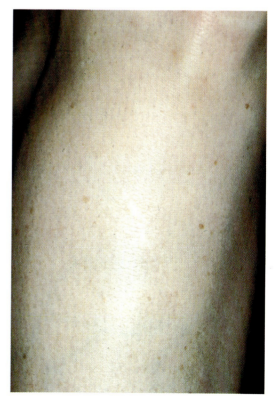

Figure 12-3c
Page 212

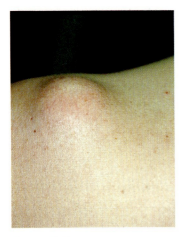

Figure 12-7a
Page 218

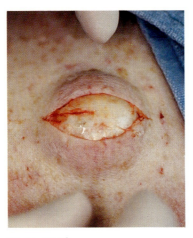

Figure 12-7b
Page 218

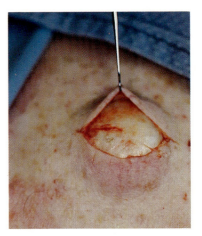

Figure 12-7c
Page 218

Figure 12-8a
Page 220

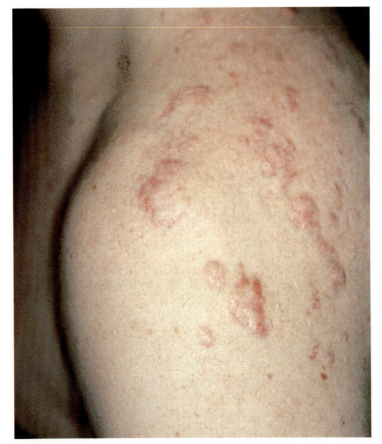

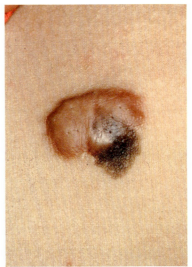

Figure 12-8b
Page 220

For complete figure caption, see the page number(s) indicated.

slippage of very fine tissue and are used for trimming grafts and cutting thin tissue such as that in a periocular location.

Scissors can be stainless steel or tungsten carbide, in which the cutting edge has a tungsten carbide insert bonded onto the scissors edges. Tungsten carbide scissors are very strong and are usually guaranteed for 5 years. Supercut scissors are also available. These black-handled scissors have a finer bevel angle at the cutting edge.

Iris scissors are probably the most common scissors used for

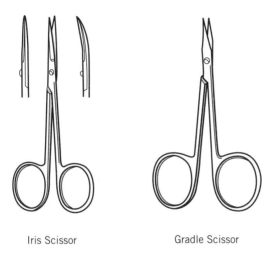

Iris Scissor

Gradle Scissor

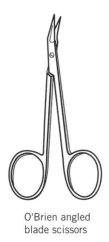

O'Brien angled
blade scissors

Figure 7-7. Surgical Scissors
Surgical scissors are available in various types and sizes. (a) Sharp tips for cutting tissue.

Surgical Instruments

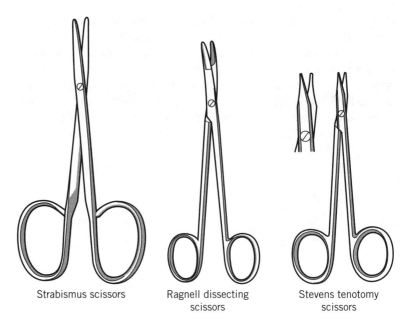

Strabismus scissors

Ragnell dissecting scissors

Stevens tenotomy scissors

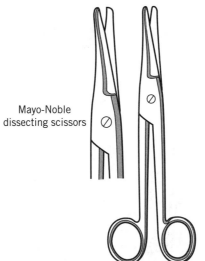

Mayo-Noble dissecting scissors

Figure 7-7. (Continued)
(b) Blunt tips for fine dissecting.

cutting tissue in skin surgery. They have sharp tips that are either straight or curved. They have relatively short handles and are easy to use for very fine, sharp dissection and cutting tissue. There are other scissors that are also commonly used for working with delicate tissue. Gradle scissors are sharp tipped and tapered to a very fine point with a gentle curve. Westcott and Castroveijo scissors operate with a spring action. Their very sharp tips come together as the handles are gently squeezed. These scissors are ideal for very delicate procedures. Sutures should not be cut with fine tissue scissors, as this may quickly dull the tips or stress and break the blades. Larger, less expensive scissors can be used to cut sutures.

Blunt-tipped instruments are typically used to undermine tissue. Longer handles are used for more extensive undermining or for freeing up larger flaps. Metzenbaum scissors are long handled and have a high handle to blade length. The resultant small blade arc makes the Metzenbaum scissors excellent for sharp or blunt dissection. The Baby Metzenbaum are considered standard undermining scissors for skin procedures. For more superficial and delicate undermining, the Steven's tenotomy scissors are excellent. Other undermining scissors include Ragnell, Shea, and Kilner scissors.

Specially designed scissors are available for removing fine sutures. Suture removal scissors have either curved or straight blades with a depression in one blade to more easily grasp the suture loop. Blunt tips help prevent accidental sticks. The 3.5 in. length is more popular. Lister scissors are the most popular bandage scissors. They come in a variety of sizes but the 5.5 in. model is most commonly used. It has angled blades and large blunt tips that easily slide under a dressing without causing damage to the underlying skin. Universal scissors are also used for removing dressings and have serrated edges and larger ring sizes that provide greater cutting power.

Of the various surgical instruments used in skin surgery, scissors require the most attention for cleaning and care. It is imperative to maintain both blade sharpness and tip approximation.

CURETTE

The curette is an instrument used very commonly by dermatologists but uncommonly by other cutaneous surgeons. Excellent for the treatment of superficial benign and malignant lesions, the curette also has great utility in defining the margins of a basal cell or squamous cell carcinoma before definitive surgical excision is done.

Curette handles can be slender or broad. The heads are usually round or oval and vary in size from 1 mm to 7 mm, typically in 1 mm gradations. The Fox curette has a slender handle with a round cutting edge. The 3 mm and 4 mm sizes are the most popular [Figure 7-8]. The Piffard curette has an oval cutting head with a heavier handle [Figure 7-8a]. It comes in small, medium, and large sizes. Smaller curettes with heads varying in size from 0.5 mm to 3 mm are used to curette small pockets of tumor or to curette small cyst walls. Commonly used small curettes are the Skeele, Heath, and Meyhoefer. Like scissors, curettes become dull and must be sharpened on a regular basis. Improper sharpening of curettes and scissors can easily ruin these instruments. It is usually best to have this service performed by a reliable vendor or use the disposable, single-use curettes.

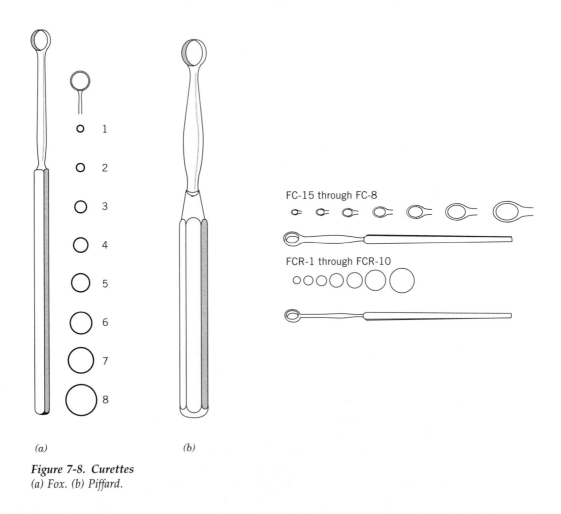

Figure 7-8. Curettes
(a) Fox. (b) Piffard.

MISCELLANEOUS INSTRUMENTS

Punch

The skin punch has been used in dermatologic surgery for many years. Developed in the late 1800s by Keyes, the original had a heavy handle, slanted sides, and a beveled cutting edge. Newer punches were developed for hair transplantation surgery with very sharp edges and a straight inner wall. These punches can be reused after sterilization but have a tendency to become dull and somewhat unpredictable with use. Disposable punches have become very popular because of convenience and their very sharp cutting edge. Cutting is exact and consistent. They are available in sizes from 1.5 mm to 6 mm. Although not reusable, disposable punches prove to be cost efficient for single biopsy procedures. The major purpose of the punch is for skin biopsies, but it can also be used to completely excise small lesions.

Chalazion Clamp

The chalazion clamp was designed for removal of chalazia around the eye, but is useful for excisions and biopsies of the mouth and tongue. The chalazion clamp handle is shaped like a forceps, but the distal tip has a solid, oval plate on one side and a ring of similar diameter on the other [Figure 7-9]. On the shaft there is a thumbscrew that, when tightened, holds the two surfaces close together, thus isolating the lesion to be removed. It provides a firm, immobile surface on which to work and also provides excellent hemostasis. The Desmarres chalazion clamp comes in three sizes: small (20 mm), medium (26 mm), and large (31 mm).

Towel Clip

A towel clip should routinely be included on every surgical tray. When draping a patient for skin surgery using sterile drapes, towel clips allow the drapes to be firmly anchored in place. The clip can also be used to secure the electrocautery handle.

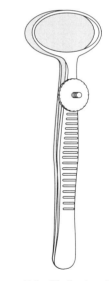

Figure 7-9. Chalazion Clamp

INSTRUMENT CARE

After investing a substantial amount of money in quality surgical instruments, it is important to take care of them in a proper fashion to ensure longevity and proper functioning. Improper care will dramatically reduce the useful life of a surgical instrument. Correct cleaning, sterilization, and packaging maintains safety and efficacy while regular lubrication and sharpening will maintain precision. Stainless steel instruments will stain and rust if not properly cared for. Never use bleach or household cleaner on surgical instruments.

Clean all instruments immediately after use [Table 7-2]. They should be rinsed in cold water to remove blood and debris. Instruments can be soaked in distilled water or a solution of neutral pH detergent. The soaking solutions need to be changed on a daily basis. Instruments should be manually cleaned vigorously with a bristled brush and detergent. Warm water can be used for the initial rinsing of the instrument, but ideally distilled water should be used for a second rinsing. This two-step rinsing will remove remnants of surgical debris as well as remove potential contaminants that may be in the normal tap water.

Alternatively, instruments may be rinsed and placed in an ultrasonic cleanser [Table 7-3]. Ultrasonic cleansers work by a process called *cavitation* in which sonic waves dislodge and clean debris. If instruments are soaked in a disinfectant, it is important to rinse these prior to ultrasonic cleaning. Ultrasonic cleaners are manufactured with rinsing and drying chambers. A 12-minute cycle is usually required. Cleaning solution should be changed daily. After instruments are thoroughly dried, they are packaged prior to sterilization. Instruments are typically placed in a wrapping material of paper or cloth. It is wise to design surgical instrument packs for commonly performed procedures such as biopsies, suture removal, shave excisions, and excisional procedures.

TABLE 7-2 Manual Cleaning Procedure

1. Inspect instruments for cracks or chips.
2. Clean instruments immediately after use.
3. Use a neutral pH solution and follow manufacturers' instructions for soaking time and mixing ratios.
4. Clean all instruments with a soft brush; never use a steel brush or scouring pad. Clean instruments in an open position and be careful to remove all debris from the box locks.
5. After cleaning thoroughly, rinse instruments in distilled water.
6. Dry instruments with clean, lint-free towels.
7. Soak in an instrument milk 30–60 seconds prior to sterilizing.

TABLE 7-3 Ultrasonic Cleaning Procedure

1. Inspect all instruments for cracks and chips.
2. Rinse off debris in tap water.
3. Use a neutral pH cleaning solution.
4. Place instruments in ultrasonic cleaner in an open position. Do not stack instruments on top of each other.
5. Follow manufacturers' instructions for the cleaning cycle time. Do not allow instruments to soak after the cycle time is completed.
6. Rinse thoroughly with distilled water.
7. Dry instruments with clean, dry, lint-free towel.
8. Soak in instrument milk 30–60 seconds prior to sterilizing.

Sterilization is defined as the process of completely destroying microbial life. Various means are available for sterilization, including dry heat, steam, chemical vapor, and gas. Gas sterilization is used in most hospital settings. In the office setting the steam sterilizer is most commonly employed. Steam under pressure kills microorganisms by coagulation of proteins. Steam sterilizers are commonly referred to as *autoclaves*. Steam autoclaves work best using distilled water. Chemical vapor sterilization uses a chemical instead of distilled water in the steam autoclave process. Popular autoclave systems are the Harvey and Ritter steam autoclaves.

Lubrication of instruments is important for proper functioning. Silicone oil compounds are used with steam sterilization autoclaves. Also, oil and water emulsions (instrument milk) effectively precoat the instruments before sterilization. These solutions may also help to prevent corrosion of instruments.

THE SURGICAL SUITE

The size, design, and number of outpatient operating rooms you maintain depends on the extent, scope, and nature of the cutaneous surgery you will perform. The doctor who performs only limited minor surgical procedures probably does not require an extensive outpatient surgical suite. On the other hand, if you perform complex closures, laser procedures, or Mohs' surgery, a more fully equipped outpatient surgical room is an absolute necessity. The design and layout of the surgical room is very important. It should be comfortable for physician, staff, and patient. It should be at least 150–200 square feet. The room must accommodate ancillary support staff and all necessary equipment, including (but not limited to) a power electric table, overhead lighting, mobile equipment stand, sink, patient dressing area, stool, electrical surgical apparatus, suction equipment, waste containers, and ample counter and storage space. The facility must be large enough to allow easy movement around the surgical table and the ceiling needs to be high enough to accommodate overhead lighting. Patients are typically anxious about surgery and, therefore, the surgical suite should have a warm and comfortable feel to it. Easy-to-clean wallpaper will help minimize the sterile feel of white walls. Artwork will give the patient something to focus on during the surgical procedure. The floor should be hard and seamless to facilitate cleaning. Window light adds to room warmth and individual temperature control is important. Music should be soothing. The use of earphones can help minimize awareness of strange surgical sounds.

Each surgical room must have a sink, preferably 18–24 inches deep. Foot pedals are very convenient for handwashing. In the same way that a house can never have enough closet space, a surgical room can never have enough cabinet and counter space. There should be easy access to instruments and supplies and adequate room to store them. If you use more than one surgical suite, it is preferable that each room be laid out in the same manner so as to decrease confusion about instrument and supply location. The quality of the cabinets will depend on what you can afford. Wood cabinets add a certain warmth, but at a cost; laminated cabinets are easiest to clean. Open cabinets or glass cabinets will allow easy visualization of supplies. Countertops should be nonporous, durable, and easy to clean.

Equipping the outpatient surgical suite is a long-term investment—don't be cheap or you will be disappointed. It is important to shop around and get several competitive bids. A well-equipped surgical room (instruments excluded) will probably cost at least $20,000. It is also important to lay out the room so that you will have easy access to the instruments and patient [Figure 7-10].

1. *Surgical table.* The operating table should be a high-quality, electric-powered table that is easily adjusted and provides for both patient and physician comfort. The table should be easily controlled by fingertip- or foot-operated panels. Multiple joints to the table allow for flexible adjustment of the back, head, and feet, as well as up or down elevation and a tilt. The tilt position will allow the patient to be placed quickly in the Trendelenburg position if necessary. Tables come in various dimensions. Wider tables accommodate larger patients while a narrow table allows easier physician access. Head rests should be comfortable; a pillow is often added for extra

comfort, especially in patients with neck problems. Detachable arm rests are invaluable when working on the lower arm and hand. Tables may come with built-in stirrups, Mayo stands, and restraint straps.

2. *Surgical chair.* At times it may be preferable for the physician to sit for certain procedures. A comfortable chair is imperative. It should be on rollers and have a pneumatic height adjustment controlled by hand or foot. The stool should have an extended back rest.

3. *Lights.* You cannot perform skilled surgery if you cannot see what you are doing. Optimal lighting cannot be stressed enough. There is a wide range of surgical lighting with a corresponding wide range of costs. The intensity of the light is expressed in foot-candles and ranges from 3,000 to 8,000. Lights are most convenient if mounted overhead, but in smaller rooms they can be wall mounted. Ceiling track lighting allows for the greatest mobility: 360 degrees and from head to foot. Lights should be installed to permit illumination at any position on the surgical table. The surgical lights should be multisource so as to minimize shadows. They should be high intensity, simple to adjust and maneuver, and with sterile handles. At times, two overhead lights can provide even better illumination, but the room needs to be large enough to accommodate both. Head-mounted single-point lights can be used for supplemental lighting

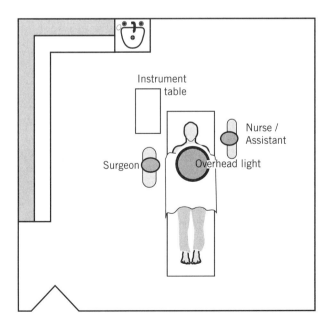

Figure 7-10. Layout
Your office surgery suite should be laid out in a fashion that permits easy access to the patient and to your instruments. It is important also to have your assistant positioned so that everyone around the patient is comfortable. Avoiding needle sticks and other accidents within the busy surgical field is critical.

and can be quite helpful when working in smaller and deeper areas, such as the mouth or ear canal.

4. *Suction.* Suction equipment is needed to control occasional profuse bleeding. Wall suction is the most powerful and desirable, but also the most expensive. Portable units (Gomco or AEROS aspirators) are commonly used. Laser vacuums can also be modified to provide excellent suction.

5. *Electrosurgical equipment.* Electrosurgical equipment provides a variety of functions including cutting, fulguration, coagulation, and desiccation. The Birtcher hyfrecator is a commonly used monopolar electrosurgical instrument available at a reasonable cost. It does *not* provide a cutting current and is used primarily for fulguration and desiccation. Electrodesiccation generally provides excellent hemostasis for small bleeding vessels. The Birtcher unit can be portable (attached to a floor stand) or wall mounted because it is relatively small and lightweight. There is fingertip control of the current and of the power setting. Tips are disposable and come both as sharp and blunt. There is no need to ground the patient. It works best in a dry surgical field and loses some efficiency in areas of heavy bleeding. In these instances, suction becomes very important.

The Bovie is a multifunctional electrosurgical instrument that allows for both coagulation and cutting. A grounding or dispersive electrode is used that is held in contact with the patient to direct current flow. Biterminal forceps allow more pinpoint coagulation by the use of two active electrodes. The Surgitron (Ellman) uses radiowave frequency and provides four different currents for cutting, cutting plus coagulation, coagulation only, and spark gap desiccation.

6. *Instrument stand.* Commonly referred to as a Mayo stand or table, the instrument stand should be sturdy, maneuverable, and adjustable. A Mayo table rests on four casters and is very stable and easily moved. A Mayo stand has two casters and generally is not as stable. The advantage of a stand is that it can be placed over the patient if desired. Instruments should be placed on the tray so that needle-stick risk will be minimized and all instruments are readily accessible (Figure 7-11).

➡ Your suite design must incorporate all OSHA and blood-borne pathogen guidelines. Waste-disposal buckets must be readily available to accommodate all contaminated materials.

7. *Waste disposal.* Kick-bucket waste containers are stainless steel buckets on wheels that are easily moved. Sharp containers should be attached to the wall, out of reach of children, wide mouthed, and puncture proof.

The Surgical Suite

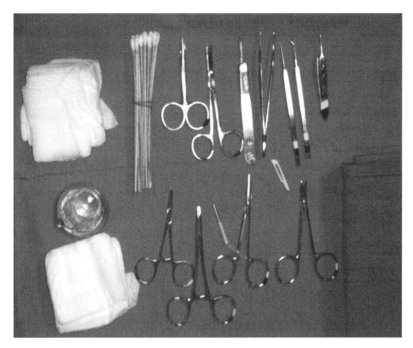

Figure 7-11. Instrument Tray
The organization of the surgical tray is critical for safety and efficiency. A medicine glass can be used to temporarily store needles, blades and other hazardous materials until the tray is disassembled.

8. *Emergency equipment—crash cart.* It is a wise practice, although not absolutely mandatory, to have a crash cart in an office surgical suite. Ideally, the crash cart should include a defibrillator (the EKG monitor can also be used for rhythm strips in nonemergency situations), as well as the appropriate equipment and drugs for advanced cardiopulmonary resuscitation. Surgical personnel should be trained in advanced cardiac life support. An oxygen tank should be available for both emergency and nonemergency situations. IV equipment should be readily available. In case of a power failure all offices should be equipped with backup support systems that include an auxiliary power source and emergency lighting.

9. *Oxygen monitor.* If patients are to be sedated, it is essential to have an oxygen monitor to provide continuous monitoring of pulse rate and oxygen saturation level. Sedated patients also require continuous blood pressure monitoring.

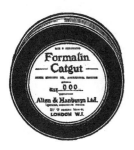
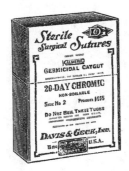
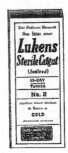
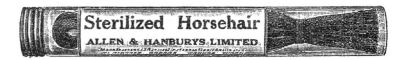
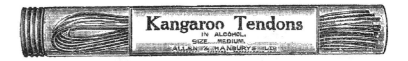
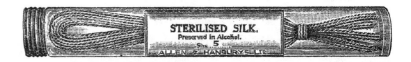
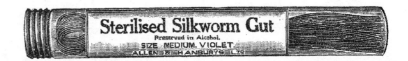

8

Wound Closure Materials

No one suture or wound closure material is ideal for all patients, at all times, or for every procedure by all surgeons. Different patients, procedures, circumstances, and personal preferences of the surgeon will dictate what type of wound closure material should be used. It is very important to learn proper surgical technique, but it is equally important to understand the proper use and selection of sutures and other wound closure materials. There is a wide array of suture materials and needles and some confusion exists due to inconsistent nomenclature by the different manufacturers. [See Table 8-1] The dermatologic surgeon should understand the basic properties of all suture materials in order to maximize the cosmetic and functional outcome for the patient.

The purpose of sutures is to maintain wound closure until the repair has matured. During the first 1–2 weeks postoperatively the intrinsic tensile strength of the wound is only approximately 7%–10%. Sutures provide support during this most vulnerable period. The use of nonabsorbable, buried, subcutaneous sutures is especially important during the first month when the wound is most at risk for dehiscence. The more superficial skin sutures will allow fine approximation of the epidermal wound edges and thus an improved cosmetic result.

In reviewing the physical characteristics and properties of suture material, it is helpful to contemplate what constitutes the "ideal" suture. It should tie easily and hold the knot securely. It should have excellent tensile strength. It should cause no adverse effects on healing and it should not promote infection or cause tissue reac-

➡ Ideal Suture Features

1. Easy to handle and tie
2. Secure knot
3. Pulls through tissue easily
4. Strong
5. Will not promote infection or tissue reactivity
6. Inexpensive

Wound Closure Materials

TABLE 8-1 Suture Material Characteristics

	Tensile Strength (Half-life in Days)	Knot Security	Ease of Handling	Tissue Reactivity
Absorbable				
Fast absorbing gut	2	low	low	med
Plain gut	4	low	low	high
Chromic gut	7	med	low	high
PDS (polydioxanone)	28	med	poor	med
Vicryl (polyglactin 910)	14	med	med	low
Dexon (polyglycolic acid)	14	med	low	low
Nonabsorbable				
Silk		high	high	high
Nylon monofilament		med	med	low
Polypropylene		low	low	low

tivity. The suture itself should come in a variety of sizes and not be too costly. There are a number of terms that help describe these properties [See Table 8-1]:

1. *Configuration* refers to whether the suture is a monofilament (single stranded) or polyfilament (braided or twisted). As a general principal, a braided suture will handle and tie more easily but can lead to an increased risk of infection due to the potential of harboring organisms between the filament strands.

2. *Knot strength* refers to the force necessary to cause a knot to slip and is directly proportional to the friction coefficient of the suture material. The more slippery the suture material, the easier it is to move through tissue, but the more likely it is that the resulting knot will slip. The advantage of greater knot strength may be offset by a suture material that has more tissue drag.

3. *Tensile strength* refers to the amount of weight that is required to break a suture divided by the cross-sectional area of the suture. Tensile strength will vary with the diameter of the suture as well as the material itself. In general, stainless steel will have the highest tensile strength followed by synthetic materials and then natural materials such as silk.

4. *Diameter* of sutures is defined in millimeters and is typically expressed in USP (United States Pharmacopeia) sizes with multiples of zeros. The smaller the cross-sectional diameter of the suture, the more zeros. For example, 6-0 Prolene (polypropylene) is narrower than 4-0 Prolene. Not all USP sizes correspond to the same diameters for the same suture material. The USP size is related to the specific

diameter necessary to produce a given tensile strength. However, the tensile strength will also be affected by the suture material. Thus, 4-0 catgut is actually a larger diameter suture than 4-0 Prolene. Diameter is also referred to as the *caliber* of the suture.

5. *Capillarity* and *fluid absorption* are characteristics that refer to the ability of a suture to absorb fluid and transfer it along the suture strand. Polyfilament sutures have greater capillarity than monofilament sutures.

6. *Elasticity* is the ability of a suture to regain its original texture, form, and length after being stretched. A highly elastic suture has the ability to allow for tissue swelling, and can be stretched so as not to cut into the swollen tissue. *Plasticity* is the ability of the suture material to retain its new length and form after it has been stretched.

7. *Memory* refers to the suture's ability to return to its former shape after it has been deformed with tying. Memory is related directly to the elasticity and plasticity of the suture material. More memory results in less knot security. A suture with lots of memory, such as prolene, will be rather stiff and will handle less well. High-memory sutures require a greater number of ties to ensure the security of the knot. Suture material with low memory, such as silk, is easy to handle and rarely becomes untied.

8. *Pliability* is a subjective term that refers to how easily a suture can be bent. The most pliable sutures are those that are braided, such as silk.

9. *Friction coefficient* refers to how easily the suture will pull through tissue. It refers to how slippery the material is. Some sutures are coated in order to decrease tissue drag. Prolene, which has a low coefficient of friction, pulls easily through tissue and allows for easy removal of the suture material 1–2 weeks later.

10. *Tissue reactivity* is the degree of foreign body inflammatory response that the suture material engenders in tissue. As a general rule, natural materials (such as catgut and silk) are much more reactive than the synthetic materials (such as nylon and polypropylene). Greater tissue reactivity can result in increased risk of wound infection with delayed healing.

ABSORBABLE SUTURES

An absorbable suture is defined as a suture that will lose most of its tensile strength within 60 days after being placed beneath the skin surface. Loss in strength does not necessarily mean that the suture will be completely absorbed. Early absorbable sutures were of animal origin (collagen) and more recent absorbable sutures are synthetic. Commonly used absorbable sutures are discussed below.

Catgut (Surgical Gut)

Although catgut has been used since the second century A.D., it is infrequently used today. It is derived from the intestinal intima of sheep or cattle. It is packaged wet in alcohol and dries quickly when exposed to air. Surgical gut is available as plain or chromic. The chromic catgut is treated with chromium salts to produce a tougher and stronger suture. The major disadvantages of catgut include poor tensile strength, high tissue reactivity, and poor knot stability. Catgut retains its useful tensile strength for only 4–5 days and has almost no tensile strength at 2 weeks. It can be ordered as fast-absorbing gut to be used as a percutaneous suture that is rapidly degraded in 4–5 days. Its primary use is for fine epidermal approximation of skin grafts and occasionally for suturing wounds on children where it may be difficult to remove sutures.

Polyglycolic Acid (Dexon)

Dexon, the first synthetic absorbable suture, was introduced in 1970 as a polymer of glycolic acid. It represented a vast improvement over catgut. Its tensile strength was good, with approximately 50% tensile strength at 2 weeks. By 1 month it has retained only 5% of its original tensile strength and is predictably totally degraded by approximately 90 days. It comes in a braided configuration to allow easier handling.

Dexon is either uncoated or coated. Coating the Dexon suture allows it to pull more easily through the tissue and permits smoother knot tying. The original coating was poloxamer 188 (Dexon Plus), but more recently a new synthetic coating of polycaprolate (Dexon Two) allows for improved handling qualities. Whereas catgut is degraded by proteolytic enzymes, Dexon is degraded by hydrolysis, which results in less of an inflammatory response.

Polyglactin 910 (Vicryl)

Vicryl was introduced in 1974 and represented the second synthetic absorbable suture. It is a braided suture copolymer of lactide and glycolide. A lubricant coating allows for easier pull through tissue. Because it is hydrolyzed, it has minimal tissue reactivity similar to Dexon. However, it is absorbed more quickly than Dexon, usually within 60 days. It has a high tensile strength, but only 8% of its tensile strength remains at 1 month.

This suture comes as white or violet. The dyed form may be visible beneath the skin surface. Occasionally there will be a clinically apparent reaction to Vicryl, which is felt as a ''lump'' underneath the incision line. This slowly resolves with time. Vicryl and Dexon both will occasionally extrude if placed close to the surface. This ''spitting stitch'' will appear on the skin surface as a small pustule. Patients may be alarmed that they have an underlying infection. This commonly will be seen at 3–4 weeks, and patients can be reassured of the benign nature of the reaction.

Polydioxanone (PDS)

This monofilament polymer was introduced in 1980. It is a polymer of polydioxanone. Its primary advantage is its prolonged tensile strength compared to Dexon or Vicryl. At 2 weeks it retains 74% of its original tensile strength, and at 4 weeks it still has 58%. It does not undergo complete absorption until 180 days. It is a good choice for an absorbable suture when prolonged wound tensile strength is needed. The major disadvantage of PDS is that it is stiffer and less pliable than Dexon or Vicryl and therefore a little more difficult to tie. Like Dexon and Vicryl, it has minimal tissue reactivity.

Polytrimethylylene Carbonate (Maxon)

Maxon is a synthetic monofilament that combines the prolonged tensile stength seen with PDS along with improved handling and tying qualities. Maxon has a tensile strength retention of 81% at 14 days and 59% at 28 days. Complete absorption occurs around 180 days. Despite this prolonged absorption, there is minimal tissue reactivity. Unlike PDS, Maxon has more supple handling with a very smooth knot tie-down.

Poliglecaprone 25 (Monocryl)

Monocryl is the newest monofilament copolymer made of glycolide and *e*-caprolactone. It maintains 60% of its tensile strength at 7 days and requires 90–100 days for complete absorption. It has only slight tissue reactivity. The major advantage of monocryl is the suppleness and ease of handling. It is the most expensive of the absorbable sutures.

NONABSORBABLE SUTURES

By definition, nonabsorbable sutures are resistant to degradation. However, the term is relative in that some of these sutures will eventually be degraded. For example, nylon is classified as a nonabsorbable suture, but it is partially degraded within 3 weeks after implantation and at 6 months it may have very little tensile strength left. The most commonly used nonabsorbable sutures are discussed here.

Silk

Silk is a natural suture material made from the natural protein filaments spun by the silk worm larva. Raw silk is white, but surgical silk is dyed black for better visibility during suturing. Silk is classified as a nonabsorbable suture but in reality will slowly absorb over many months when it is buried in subcutaneous tissue. Silk handles extremely well and is perhaps the easiest suture to tie.

The major disadvantage of silk is its very low tensile strength and greater tissue reactivity. It produces more of an inflammatory reaction in tissue than any other suture except catgut. Because silk is a braided suture, its high capillarity increases the risk of infection. Because of the tissue handling properties of silk, as well as its low memory and ability to lie flat, it is extremely useful on mucosal surfaces, intertriginous areas, and around the eyelids. Silk is not likely to tear tissue because it is very soft.

Nylon

Nylon, introduced in 1940, represented the first synthetic nonabsorbable suture. It is probably the most widely used nonabsorbable suture for cutaneous surgery. Its popularity is due to its minimal tissue reactivity and its relatively high tensile strength, along with a relatively low cost. Its major disadvantage is its stiffness and memory, requiring an increased number of knot throws to secure the knot. Nylon does come as a braided polyfilament suture, which gives it more pliability and makes it easier to handle but at an increased cost. Monofilament nylon comes in black, green, or clear.

Clear buried nylon sutures are sometimes used in an attempt to prevent scar spread because they retain their tensile strength for a very long time.

Polypropylene (Prolene, Surgilene)

Polypropylene (Prolene, Surgilene) is a plastic suture formed by the polymerization of propylene. Polypropylene is a flexible monofilament with fair to good tensile strength although it is not as strong as nylon. Its major advantage is the smoothness of its surface, which results in very little tissue drag and easy pull through tissue. It makes suture removal relatively painless. It is excellent for running intradermal sutures. Polypropylene is also very plastic and therefore stretches and remains deformed with wound and tissue swelling. There is very little cutting through the tissue and very little inflammatory tissue reaction. A disadvantage of Prolene is its memory and smoothness, which compromises knot security. Prolene costs more than nylon.

Polyesters (Dacron, Mersilene, Ethibond)

Polyester sutures are polymers that are formed as nylon by condensation polymerization. These sutures are braided polyfilaments and therefore handle very well. They also have a very high tensile strength and are stronger than either nylon or polypropylene. Their one disadvantage is a relatively rough surface that produces drag through tissue and when knots are tied. Some polyester sutures have lubricant coatings of silicone or polybutilate to produce a smoother surface. Polyester sutures and polypropylene sutures will maintain their tensile strength forever and will not resorb. Thus, they are sometimes recommended for permanent buried sutures. The effectiveness of polyesters in preventing scar spread is unknown.

Polybutester (Novafil)

Polybutester is the newest of the nonabsorbable sutures and is a thermoplastic copolymer. It is a highly elastic suture with the capacity to stretch 50% of its length. This elasticity allows for elongation of the suture when wound edema occurs and maintenance of tension on the wound when the edema recedes. Because it is a monofilament, there is very little tissue inflammatory reaction. Like polypropylene, it has a slippery smooth surface and very little tissue drag.

Wound Closure Materials

NEEDLES

The purpose of the needle is to bring the suture through the tissue with minimal trauma and prevent tearing of the skin. Unfortunately, needle nomenclature is confusing and inconsistent. However, it is important to be knowledgeable about needles because of cosmetic and cost concerns. The needle is made of high-quality stainless steel and is often the reason for the higher cost of a given suture material. The final needle selection will depend on the tissue thickness, tissue accessibility of the wound, and the size of the selected suture material.

A needle is composed of three parts: the shank, body, and point [Figure 8-1]. Most needles used for cutaneous surgery have a swaged shank in which the suture is placed inside a hollowed end. The metal is then crimped. Keep in mind that the largest diameter of the needle is the shank and it is this diameter which determines the size of the suture track and not the suture calibre itself.

The body of the needle is either round, triangular, or flattened. Round bodies gradually taper to a point. Triangular bodies have cutting edges along three sides. "P" and "PS" needles are flattened

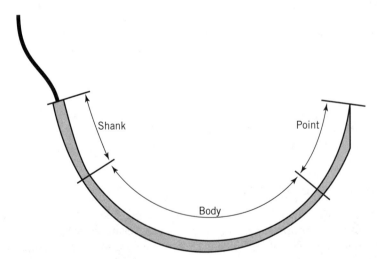

Figure 8-1. Needle Anatomy
The needle should be held approximately one-third of the way from the back end to allow for proper rotation of the needle through the arc using simple wrist motion.

at the top and bottom and the newer "PC" needles are also flat along the sides.

The needle point is one of three types: conventional cutting, reverse cutting, or round with a tapered point [Figure 8-2]. Conventional cutting needles have the cutting edge facing the inside of the curvature, whereas reverse cutting needles have a flat edge facing the inside of the curvature with the cutting edge toward the side. Reverse cutting needles have the theoretical advantage of minimizing the risk of cutting through tissue.

The precision cosmetic (PC) needle is a conventional cutting needle with a narrow, sharply honed point that is excellent for delicate cosmetic work. Other needles that work well on important cosmetic areas are the PS, PRE, and P needles. F, S, and CE needles have larger reverse cutting tips and are used primarily on thicker skin [Table 8-2]. Most needles used in cutaneous surgery have a curvature of ⅜ in. (arc of 135 degrees) and a few are ½ in. The needle curvature length will vary from 11 mm to 19 mm.

When ordering sutures, it is important to specify the size of the suture, the suture material, the size and type of needle, the suture color, and the length of the suture. Keep in mind that the type of

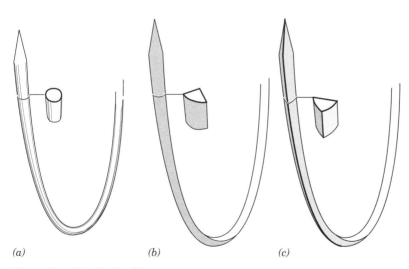

(a) (b) (c)

Figure 8-2. Needle Profiles
Advancing edges of the needle are demonstrated here. The reverse cutting needle is the most commonly used in skin surgery procedures. (a) Conventional cutting (b) Precision cosmetic (c) Reverse cutting.

Wound Closure Materials

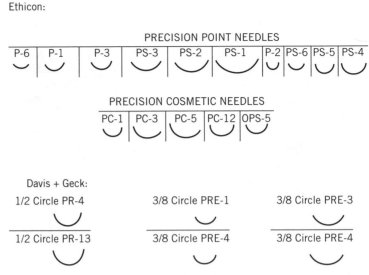

Figure 8-3. Needle Nomenclature by Manufacturers

needle will be the most important cost factor. In general suture calibres of 5-0 and 6-0 are used primarily on the face and neck and 4-0 and 5-0 are typically used on the trunk and extremities. Wounds under greater tension will require 3-0 or 4-0. There are several companies that produce sutures including Ethicon and Davis and Geck so it is important to become familiar with the quality of their needles and sutures. [Figure 8-3].

TABLE 8-2 Needle Nomenclature

FS	for skin
P	plastic
PC	precision cosmetic
PS	plastic surgery
CE	cutting
PRE	premium

STAPLES

Staples are made of stainless steel and have the advantage of highest tensile strength with very low tissue reactivity. They are used most commonly in areas of significant tension (scalp) and provide excellent wound eversion with minimal cross-hatch scarring. A major advantage of staples is that they can be placed faster and with less effort than sutures. Staples are also less likely to become infected because they do not form a complete track from one wound edge to the other. A disadvantage of staples is that they may be uncomfortable for the patient. Proper placement of staples may be difficult and requires experience. There are specially designed staple extractors but patients still generally complain of more discomfort when staples are removed compared with the removal of regular sutures.

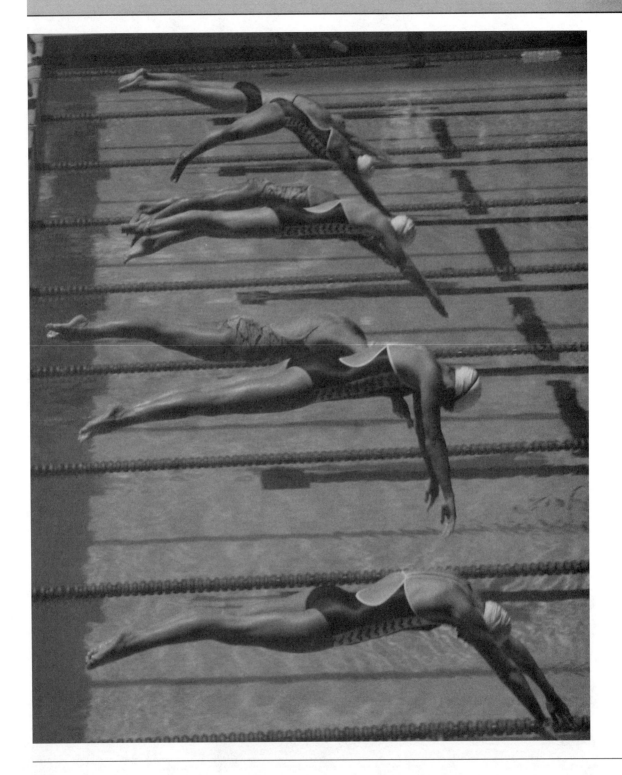

9

Patient Preparation

Patient preparation is probably the single most important step one can pursue to assure a successful overall surgical outcome. Skill is a function of the operator and intrinsic healing is a function of uncontrollable genetics. Preparing the patient for the procedure he or she is about to undergo and controlling as many of the variables as possible is one way for the surgeon to effect a desirable outcome and compensate for those factors beyond his or her control. While judgment is the father of successful surgery, planning is the midwife. Included in good planning is the clinical diagnosis and the need for surgery, the medical history, the drug history, the infectious history, the healing history, previous responses to anesthetics, evaluation of anxiety level, an appraisal of the patient's lifestyle and activity level, and a determination about whether the patient understands the procedure and all the attendant risks.

INDICATIONS

Whether performing a biopsy or a complete lesional excision, it is important to be certain that the procedure itself is indicated. A biopsy, of course, is done to make a histologic diagnosis. An excision is done either for a similar reason or for therapeutic purposes, to remove a malignant lesion or to evaluate in its entirety a lesion that is of concern. In the realm of skin surgery, many procedures may be considered elective, and as such the risks of the procedure must be balanced against the potential benefits of performing it.

In general, skin surgery is substantially less risky than other forms of routine surgery. The ultimate downside is transient infection, bleeding, or a permanent unsatisfactory cosmetic result. Rarely, however, do the adverse effects associated with skin surgery have a long-term impact that directly or indirectly affects quality of life. Nonetheless, an unsatisfactory scar resulting from an unnecessary excision that the patient was not convinced was necessary can become a source of constant frustration, like a burr stuck inside a sock on a mountain hike. No matter how much one tries to eliminate fragments of the burr, the discomfort still seems to persist. In general, when skin cancer is suspected, biopsy or excision is medically indicated. The removal of a benign-appearing nevus on the face, however, is purely cosmetic and cannot in any way be construed as a nonelective procedure.

MEDICAL HISTORY

It is essential to obtain a complete medical history and review of systems at the time of consultation. [Table 9.1]. The medical history for skin surgery is more focused than what might be obtained for an annual physical examination. Figure 9-1 demonstrates the patient intake form used in our practice (DJL). Aside from the routine questions, we attempt to be as specific as possible about the reason for presentation. This, filled out in the patient's own hand, confirms at a later date the reason for the patient's presentation if any questions arise subsequent to procedures that are performed.

A medication history is important. It provides information about the use of penicillamine, which can affect healing, as well as prednisone and other agents that inhibit collagen growth and could be expected to increase the incidence of wound dehiscence or unsatisfactory results. Similarly, many patients use aspirin as cardiac and stroke prophylaxis and this should be elicited. Very often patients do not consider aspirin a medication and may not list it. For this reason it is important to specifically question the patient about use of this agent or other antiplatelet medications available over the counter. It is helpful to list the agents by brand name, as patients may not otherwise recognize them. The effect of aspirin on platelet adhesion lasts for approximately 10 days, permanently affecting the platelet for the duration of its lifespan. That is, it is eliminated only when the platelet dies. The other nonsteroidal anti-inflammatory

Medical History

TABLE 9-1 Review of Systems in Cutaneous Surgery

System	Problem	Perioperative Problem
Endocrine	Thyrotoxicosis	↑ Cardiac sensitivity to epinephrine
	Pregnancy	Effects of local anesthetics on fetus
	Diabetes	↑ Time of wound healing (if poorly controlled); infection
Pulmonary	Emphysema	↑ Toxicity of local anesthetics (caused by respiratory acidosis)
Renal	Renal failure	↑ Toxicity of local anesthetics; adjustment of antibiotics
	Hypokalemia	↑ Cardiac arrhythmia with epinephrine
Cardiac	Heart failure	↑ Toxicity of local anesthetics
	Arrhythmia	↑ Toxicity of epinephrine
	Pacemakers	Interference by electromagnetic radiation
Gastrointestinal	Cirrhosis	↑ Toxicity to anesthetics
		↑ Bleeding
	Hepatitis	Possible inoculation
Hematopoietic	Bleeding disorder	↑ Bleeding or hematoma
	Anticoagulation	↑ Bleeding
	Infection other than operative site	↑ Wound infection
	Keloids	↑ Scar formation
Central nervous system	Neurosis	Noncooperative or unpredictable patient
	Psychosis	
	Cryoglobulinemia	Cold (for example, from liquid N_2) could cause precipitation of cryoglobulins
Miscellaneous	Pseudocholintesterase deficiency	↓ Plasma clearance of ester anesthetics
	Herpes simplex (recurrent)	Herpes simplex reactivation
	AIDS	Possible inoculation

Source: Adapted from Bennett, R. G., 1988, *Fundamentals of Cutaneous Surgery*, Mosby, St. Louis, MO.

agents effect a reversible inhibition of platelet adhesion and the effect usually is lost after 3–5 hours. It has been our experience, however, that patients continue to bleed if they have been taking substantial amounts of nonsteroidal anti-inflammatory medications.

It is also important to take note of whether the patient is on any psychotropic medications, as these will certainly affect your threshold for performing elective cosmetic procedures. Obtain a history of past infections, either in the surgical setting or otherwise. The patient may be predisposed to infection and you may choose to prophylax. Infectious diseases that may be transmitted to those in the operative field must be identified and documented. Universal precautions should be closely followed.

➥ Never clean a surgical field with alcohol immediately prior to surgery or biopsy. Alcohol is highly flammable and electrocautery can ignite a flash of fire on the skin, leading to a serious burn.

Yale University Department of Dermatology
Patient Medical History

Name _____ Age _____ Date of Birth _____ Date _____

(If patient is a minor):
Parent/Guardian Name: _____

INSURANCE:

Do you live alone? Yes ❏ No ❏
In case of emergency please contact: _____ Phone: _____

Home Address: _____
City _____ State _____ Zip _____
Alternate address (seasonal): _____

City _____ State _____ Zip _____
Daytime Phone _____ Evening Phone _____
Education (highest level) _____ Occupation _____

Who referred you to our practice? Physician (see below) Yes ❏ Other: _____

	Referring Physician	Family Physician/Pediatrician
Name		
Street		
City		
Phone Number		

MEDICAL HISTORY

Do you have or have you ever had any of the following conditions?

CONDITION	Y	N	CONDITION	Y	N	CONDITION	Y	N
DIABETES			ASTHMA			HEART DISEASE		
HIGH BLOOD PRESSURE			RHEUMATIC FEVER			CHEST PAIN		
ARTIFICIAL VALVE/JOINT			STROKE			PNEUMONIA		
HEPATITIS			IMMUNE SUPPRESSION			KIDNEY DISEASE		
GLAUCOMA			EMPHYSEMA			CANCER		
SEIZURES			ORGAN TRANSPLANT					

PLEASE TURN OVER FOR MORE INFORMATION TO BE COMPLETED

Figure 9-1. Patient Intake Form
The patient's past medical history, allergies, and related medical information are best obtained from the patient and in the patient's own hand. An intake form can be modified to accommodate special needs.

Medical History

List any past illness or surgery for which you were hospitalized. List with approximate date, place, type, and surgeon.

OPERATION	YEAR	OPERATION	YEAR

List and describe any ALLERGIES to medications or other substances.

_____

List any current medications. Please include all prescription and non-prescription drugs.

MEDICATION	HOW OFTEN	MEDICATION	HOW OFTEN	MEDICATION	HOW OFTEN

Are you currently taking aspirin or empirin? YES ❏ NO ❏
Do you take any cortisone (steroid) drug? YES ❏ NO ❏ DON'T KNOW ❏
    If yes, what type _____

Do you use tobacco? Now_____ Amount per day_____ Number of years_____
Did you use tobacco in the past? Yes ❏ No ❏   Date stopped _____
How much alcohol do you consume each week? _____ What type? _____
Have you ever had a blood transfusion? YES ❏ NO ❏ If yes, when _____
Weight_____ Any recent weight loss? YES ❏ NO ❏ If yes, how much?_____
Over what period of time?_____

What is the reason for your visit today?
_____

If you are here for an evaluation of skin cancer, please answer the following questions:
1.   Where is your skin lesion (skin cancer) located? _____
2.   When did you first notice this condition? _____
3.   Has your skin cancer been treated by a physician in the past? YES ❏ No ❏

     If yes, type of treatment and date _____

Signature: Date:

A history about past healing is very important and useful. Patients will often state that they form keloids and then point to a flat hypopigmented spread scar on the knee or other area. It is important to explain to the patient that these scars do not represent keloids or hypertrophic scars but, in fact, are well healed and reflect the spreading that normally occurs in areas of tension. It is important to discuss with patients the nature of scarring and what you mean by the term, so that should there be an untoward result down the road, they will have a better understanding. This is especially true when operating on areas that yield poor results such as the shoulders, back, and legs.

Ask specific questions about possible allergies to local anesthesia. Although true allergic reactions to local anesthesia is extremely rare, it is possible to have an allergic reaction to the common amide anesthetics. Such anesthetics include Novocain. It is unfortunate that the term *Novocain* is used to describe local anesthesia in much the same way Kleenex is used to describe facial tissues. In fact, Novocain is rarely used and lidocaine is the anesthetic of choice. Reactions to lidocaine are very rare. Often, patients will state that they developed a racing heart or shakiness. This was likely due to epinephrine, and in this setting one may well choose to minimize the use of epinephrine or eliminate it completely.

PATIENT EVALUATION

It is axiomatic that physicians evaluate patient anxiety on a servo basis. However, it is especially important to do so before undertaking any form of skin surgery. Although the *an*-esthesia that is obtained with chemical compounds is essential for surgery, *talk*-esthesia is equally important for preparing the patient for the procedure he or she is about to undergo.

Learning about the patient's daily activities and interests is beneficial in follow-up when you can continue to build on the doctor–patient relationship by indicating to the patient the interesting tidbits that you recall. Use this conversation opportunity to evaluate the patient's lifestyle and activity level. This is important since the first question patients will ask when they return to have sutures out, or even as soon as you are finished tying the last knot, is, "When can I resume my normal activity?" In many cases patients are tennis players, joggers, or swimmers and are eager not to interrupt a daily activity that has become an integral part of their life. You must realize that by performing surgery and limiting their activity, you are interfering directly with an aspect of their life that they consider important—in some cases even critical. Be sensitive and devise a means of performing your surgery so that there is minimal interference.

We permit patients to resume regular activity one week after sutures have been removed from the face. This is usually at 3–5 days after surgery. When wounds have been closed on the back or extremities, the deep sutures, of course, stay in place until dissolved and the superficial sutures, if any, are removed no later than 7 days after surgery. If the area is one of high tension, we ask that the patient minimize activity for a total of 10–14 days after surgery. However, this advice must be tempered by the level of eagerness on the part of the patient. Very often, patients are quite happy to take the risk of having a spread or open wound in return for being able to continue to jog on a regular basis.

Informed consent is, of course, an important aspect of preparation, increasingly so in our litigious times. Chapter 13 discusses medical-legal issues in greater detail including informed consent and legal aspects of performing surgery. Suffice it to say that the consultation should be used as an opportunity to discuss the surgery with the patient and document informed consent. When the surgery is performed on cosmetically important areas, we will invariably take a hand mirror and have the patient identify the site that he or she believes we should work on and we will then confirm it. In addition, we will then demonstrate to the patient what the wound size will be as well as the length of the linear repair. We detail this either with the end of a wooden applicator or even mark it out with a Sharpie pen. In this way there is little room for the almost universal response when the patient sees the suture line after surgery: "I didn't think the scar would be so big." Because the patient presents with a small 5 mm lesion, he or she is unprepared for the 1.5–2 cm linear scar. A review of the geometry is often necessary so that the patient understands that you have done as minimal a procedure as possible.

Remember that a scar is permanent and have a brief discussion with the patient about the difference between what a physician means by the use of the word *scar* and what the patient means by this word. We always emphasize that it is not the length of the scar that is important, but whether it is noticeable or not. Many short scars are unsightly because they are red or hypertrophic, whereas more lengthy linear scars are often so skillfully done and so well healed that they are minimally noticeable. Patients invariably understand this point and you will save yourself much anxiety later on if time is taken to represent this to the patient. In cases where it is suspected that the patient has difficulty comprehending all that is being discussed, it is not a bad idea to diagram the procedure on

➡ Have a mirror handy in all rooms and have the patient identify the specific lesion of concern prior to anesthetizing and removing.

PERMISSION FOR OPERATION OR SPECIAL PROCEDURE

NAME
ADDRESS
BIRTH DATE

SECTION "A"

Date _____, 19_____ Time _____ A.M. P.M.

The general purpose, potential benefits, possible hazards and inconveniences of _____
_____
(Specify Operation or Special Procedure)
have been explained to my satisfaction by Dr. _____ and alternatives have been discussed. The risks and benefits of the procedure have been explained and I understand them. I hereby consent to the performance of the operation or special procedure named above under his/her direction with whatever anesthesia, treatment, dressing, medication or transfusion is necessary upon _____
under his or her direction. (Myself of name of patient)

OPTIONAL

I authorize the Hospital and its Pathology section to preserve for diagnostic, scientific or teaching purposes or otherwise dispose of tissue, body parts, blood and/or body fluids removed as a result of the procedure authorized above. If the material is to be used for scientific or educational purposes, pertinent, anonymous medical information may be released with the specimen. I hereby relinquish all right, title and interest to the tissue, body parts, blood and/or body fluid, regardless of its ultimate use or disposition.

I further authorize my physician to do whatever may be necessary in the event that any unforeseen conditions arise during the course of the operation or procedure.

Signed _____
(Patient or person authorized to consent for patient)

PHYSICIAN'S NOTE

I have informed _____ of the general purpose, potential benefits, possible hazards
(Patient/Relative/Guardian)
and inconvenience of the above procedure to be performed under my direction, and alternative methods of treatment have been discussed.

ADDITIONAL PHYSICIAN COMMENTS _____
_____
_____
_____
_____
_____

Source: Adapted from Yale. New Haven Hospital, New Haven, CT

Signature of Responsible Physician

the chart in front of the patient. You then have a written record of the fact that you discussed the issues in detail with the patient, which contributes to documentation of informed consent.

A standard informed consent form is used [Figure 9-2]. It should be noted that in some jurisdictions a separate release for the use of photographs is required if such photographs, for teaching or publication purposes, can readily identify the patient.

PROPHYLAXIS

No topic presents more controversy in skin surgery than the use of prophylactic antibiotics. As patients live longer, an increasing number present with prosthetic joints, artificial heart valves, and other prostheses. In addition, with improved diagnostic techniques, it is our impression that a greater number of patients carry a diagnosis of mitral valve prolapse for which someone has told them at some point along the way that they must receive antibiotics before dental work.

The need to use prophylactic antibiotics to prevent the development of endocarditis from transient bacteremia is initially evaluated by asking the patient whether he or she normally has to take antibiotics for dental work. If the patient answers "Yes," determine what the reason is.

Although there are no well-defined guidelines for the use of prophylactic antibiotics for clean skin surgery, the literature suggests that they are not needed except in the presence of a mechanical prosthetic heart valve. However, transient bacteremia has been documented following clean skin surgery and there have been cases of patients developing clinically significant bacteremia and endocarditis following skin biopsy. The standard of care has not been clearly established in this area. Although one would be on solid scientific ground not to provide prophylactic antibiotics except in the case of prosthetic heart valve or any type of condition for which antibiotics

➥ Place a patch of occlusive dressing over your repair. This will allow patients to shower, swim, and continue other activities.

Figure 9-2. Consent Form
The purpose of a medical consent form is to document that you have communicated with the patient the risks and benefits of the procedure, the alternative therapies, and that you have answered all of the patients questions. As long as this information is contained in the consent form that you use, it should meet all legal standards. You must be able to document that you had a meaningful and useful discussion with the patient about the nature of the condition and the procedure performed to diagnose or correct it. Source: Adapted from Yale-New Haven Hospital form, New Haven, CT.

TABLE 9-2 Endocarditis Prophylaxis

Agent	Preop Dose	Postop Dose
Dicloxacillin	2 gr po 1 hour preop	1 gr po 6 hrs postop
or		
Cephalexin	1 gr po 1 hour preop	500 mp po 6 hours postop
or		
For penicillin allergy:		
Erythromycin Ethylsuccinate	800 mg po 2 hours preop	400 mg po 6 hours postop
Erythromycin stearate	1 gr po 2 hrs preop	500 mg po 6 hours postop
Clindamycin	300 mg po	150 mg po 6 hour postop
Vancomycin	500 mg IV	250 mg IV 6 hour postop

are taken before dental work, for an unclean skin surgery procedure, it is always best to balance the risk of antibiotics and the benefits to the patient. It is not unreasonable to provide prophylactic antibiotics when there is a question about the risk of developing bacteremia and endocarditis. This is especially the case if a long procedure is anticipated. Prophylactic antibiotics are only given for skin biopsy (shave or punch) when there is an indication for prophylactic antibiotic use based on the American Heart Association indications.

Although there are no clear-cut guidelines for prophylaxis in patients who are at risk for endocarditis and have clean skin wounds, it is generally best to take a cautious approach. If patients are required to take prophylactic antibiotics for dental work you should consider prophylaxing prior to skin surgery. Prophylaxis should effectively cover staphylococcal organisms. See Table 9-2 for a detailed list of available regimens.

The use of prophylactic antibiotics in patients with prosthetic joints is an even more controversial area. Well-regarded orthopedists have lined up on either side of the debate. It is best to discuss this issue with several local orthopedists and obtain a consensus opinion. Alternatively, you may consult each time with the patient's specific orthopedist. Practically speaking, this can have a deleterious impact on your surgery schedule, as you may choose to perform surgery at the time the patient is there and the need to provide prophylactic antibiotics requires an oral dose with a subsequent 1 hour waiting period or an intravenous dose, which itself is more complicated in the office setting.

Antibiotics are routinely prescribed in specific circumstances. The risk of developing resistant strains is minimal compared to the

TABLE 9-3 Antibiotic Prophylaxis for Wound Infection in Compromised Patients

Agent	1 Hour Preop Dose	6 Hours postop Dose
Dicloxacillin	1 gr po	500 mg po
Cephalexin	1 gr po	500 mp po
For penicillin allergy:		
Clindamycin	300 mg po	150 mg po

added benefit of prescribing a short 5–7 day course of antibiotics. Erythromycin is used when patients are penicillin allergic, but our drug of choice is cephalexin [Table 9-3]. Some patients are at higher risk for postoperative infection and should be treated. Diabetics, the immune-suppressed and patients with infection at other sites should be treated preventatively. Treatment one hour before surgery has been shown to decrease the incidence of infection. It has been our experience that healing is significantly improved when a short course of antibiotics is prescribed after surgery as well.

PACEMAKERS

It is important to know whether or not a patient has a pacemaker as you may need to use electrocautery to obtain hemostasis. Although pacemakers implanted since 1990 have well-manufactured filters that prevent extraneous electrical currents from resetting them, when a patient presents with a demand pacemaker it is especially important to use the electrocautery cautiously. Because both unipolar and bipolar electrocautery devices can be problematic, it is necessary to use 1-second bursts only. If there is concern about the patient's pacemaker status, it is advisable to contact the cardiologist responsible for the pacemaker and obtain his or her opinion. Similarly, the cardiologist may want to see the patient after the procedure to reevaluate the pacemaker.

BLOOD THINNERS

As the population ages it appears that more individuals are placed on warfarin (Coumadin). Atrial fibrillation was formerly the most

➡ Leg wounds heal best when natural dependent swelling is minimized. An ace bandage, applied daily and continued for 2 weeks after sutures are removed, will enable your patient to continue regular activity and speed healing.

Patient Preparation

YALE SCHOOL OF MEDICINE
DERMATOLOGIC AND LASER SURGERY UNIT

EXCISIONAL WOUND CARE INSTRUCTIONS

The DRESSING should remain in place for 24 hours. If the dressing comes loose before then, retape it carefully.

PAIN: Postoperative pain is usually minimal. Extra-strength Tylenol, two tablets every 4 hours, usually relieves any pain you may have.

BLEEDING: Careful attention has been given to your wound to prevent bleeding. The dressing you have on is a pressure dressing and will also help to prevent bleeding.

You may notice a small amount of blood on the edges of the dressing the first day and this is NORMAL. *Relax and limit your physical activity the first 48 hours after surgery.* Keep your head elevated for 48 hours if the surgery was on the face or scalp.

If bleeding seems persistent and soils the dressing, apply firm, steady pressure over the dressing with gauze for 15 minutes by the clock. This usually is adequate treatment. If bleeding still persists, call our office at _____. After hours, the dermatologist on call will return your call.

WOUND CARE: The suture line should be cleansed daily with tap water. You may gently loosen these crusts with a cotton swab. Pat dry. The first day, the wound may be tender and may bleed slightly or seep a small amount of clear fluid. For stubborn crusting, place a gauze, wet with tap water, over the wound for 5 minutes to soak and loosen the debris.

Apply a thin layer of Polysporin ointment over the wound. Cover the wound with Telfa (nonstick) dressing or a gauze pad and a piece of paper tape. It is important to keep the wound *covered.*

You may shower after 24 hours and allow the wound to get wet; however, do not let the forceful stream of the shower hit the wound directly.

You will return to our office for suture removal by Anne, Diana, Kristina or Sandy.

APPEARANCE: There may be swelling and bruising around the wound, especially near the eyes. For your comfort, you may apply warm, moist soaks to the bruises a few times a day, starting the third day after surgery. The area may remain numb for several weeks or even months. You may also experience periodic sharp pains near the wound as it heals.

The suture line will be dark pink at first and the edges of the wound will be reddened. This will lighten up day by day and will be less tender. If the wound becomes increasingly inflamed, warm, drains a puslike substance, or if you evelop a fever or chills, please call our office immediately.

Figure 9-3. Excisional Wound-Care Instructions
These wound-care instructions are presented for information. There are many different protocols that are followed. It is often helpful to review the wound-care instructions with the patient at the time of consultation and certainly right after the surgery. Source: D. Glassman, R.N., K. Kline, R.N. and A. McKeown, R.N.

WOUND CARE INSTRUCTIONS FOR GRANULATING WOUNDS

The DRESSING should remain in place for 24 hours. If the dressing comes loose before then, retape it carefully.

PAIN: Postoperative pain is usually minimal. Extra-strength Tylenol, two tablets every 4 hours, usually relieves any pain you may have.

BLEEDING: Careful attention has been given to your wound to prevent bleeding. The dressing you have on is a pressure dressing and will also help to prevent bleeding. You may notice a small amount of blood on the edges of the dressing the first day and this is NORMAL. *Relax and limit your physical activity the first 48 hours after surgery.*

If bleeding occurs and soils the dressing, apply firm steady pressure over the dressing with gauze for 15 minutes. This usually is adequate treatment. In the rare instance when bleeding persists, call us at _____.

WOUND CARE: Your wound will be granulating (growing in) over the next several weeks. Careful and meticulous wound care will help you attain a nicer, faster result. There are four different types of wound care for granulating wounds. The wound care you will follow is the one checked below:

☐ Twice daily for 5 days, and then once a day, cleanse the wound with tap water. DO NOT be afraid to wipe the wound carefully and cleanse away crusts and any drainage that may be present. The wound may be tender and may bleed slightly the first day. It may seep fluid the first few days. *Your wound will heal better if all crusts and scabs are removed.* For stubborn crusting, place a gauze wet with water over the wound for 5 minutes to soak and loosen debris. Pat dry. Reapply a pressure dressing if the wound is lightly bleeding.

☐ Apply a thin layer of *Polysporin* over the wound and cover the wound with a Telfa nonstick dressing, or a piece of gauze and paper tape. It is important to keep the wound *covered*. Do not allow it to be exposed to air.

You may shower and allow the wound to get wet; however, do not let the forceful stream of the shower hit the wound directly.

Figure 9-4. Granulating Wound Care
When wounds are allowed to heal by second intention, the results can often be excellent. Most wounds take from 3 to 4 weeks to heal completely depending on size and location. If patients are prepared properly, they can function during this period extremely well. It is important, however, to provide them with detailed instructions. There are many variations on the theme and it is best to develop your own approach. One should not allow the wounds to dry out from exposure to air. Source: D. Glassman, R.N., K. Kline, R.N. and A. McKeown, R.N.

> WOUND CARE INSTRUCTIONS FOR GRANULATING WOUNDS/PAGE TWO
>
> ☐ SILVADENE—After cleansing the wound with warm water, pat dry and apply a layer "like icing on a cake" of Silvadene to the wound. Make sure all the wound edges are coated with Silvadene. Then cover with nonstick dressing and paper tape. The Silvadene may ooze and liquify a little. This is normal. Just use a gauze to dab any excess. You will use the Silvadene daily from 1–2 weeks after which time you will use Polysporin ointment for 2 weeks and Vaseline after that until the wound is healed. Remember to always keep the wound covered.
>
> ☐ DUODERM—Change the Duoderm dressing every 2 days. If there is excess drainage from the wound, you may have to change it every day. Drainage is normal for a healing wound and it is not cause for concern. The amount of the Duoderm dressing used varies for each patient. You will be instructed on this the day of surgery.
>
> APPEARANCE: There may be swelling and bruising around the wound, especially near your eyes. For your comfort, you may apply ice over the bandage and near the wound site for 10 minutes every hour for about the first 48 hours.
>
> After a couple of days, your granulating wound will be light pinkish-yellow. This will lighten over the next couple of weeks and gradually become flesh colored. The edges of the wound will be pink at first and tender, fading after a couple of days. If the edges remain red and sore, or if the wound begins to drain pus, please notify our office (_____).
>
> The area may remain numb and be mildly itchy. You may also experience periodic pains around the wound as part of the healing process.
>
> If you have any questions, please call us at _____. We want you to feel as comfortable as possible.

Figure 9-4. Continued

common indication for warfarin, but now phlebitis, recurrent thrombosis, transient ischemic attack and stroke are increasingly the basis for which patients are anticoagulated with the drug. Antiplatelet therapy with aspirin or similar compounds are pervasive in practice. Because bleeding is one of the most common complications of skin surgery, it is important to evaluate the patient's bleeding status, confirm his or her need to be on a blood thinner, and make any appropriate adjustments. Again, consultation with the treating physician is advantageous. Remarkably, most patients on Coumadin do not have a significantly prolonged prothrombin time and rarely get into trouble with bleeding. More often, bleeding complications are noted in patients on aspirin who have a prolonged bleeding time. If aspirin can be discontinued, it should be stopped 10 days prior to surgery and may be resumed, depending on the nature of the case, 1–2 days after surgery. Coumadin, on the other hand, can be discontinued 1–2 days before surgery and resumed the day after.

We have not yet had any patients develop thrombotic events as a result of manipulation of the normal blood-thinning regimen, although this remains a distinct possibility. Obviously, in high-risk patients the possibility of stroke must be balanced against the risk of bleeding at a superficial skin excision site. Excellent hemostasis and optimal suturing techniques can compensate well for any blood thinning that is present. There is always the alternative of allowing a particular wound to heal by second intention. The minimization of undermining and disruption of normal tissue further reduces the risk of bleeding and the patient will likely heal without complications.

DRESSINGS

Patient preparation includes obtaining all the information and conveying all the necessary data prior to the procedure, but it also includes patient preparation for the postoperative period [Figures 9-3 and 9-4]. For this reason, we normally demonstrate the placement of the dressing to the patient or to the spouse or friend who will be caring for the wound. This minimizes confusion concerning wound care. A detailed plan for follow-up is made.

It is important, amongst the materials that are provided to the patient at the time of discharge, to ensure that the patient understands how to reach you with questions or problems. It is a good practice to provide your home number to patients about whom you are concerned. It is unusual to be called about matters for which you would not have wanted to be reached directly. In addition, by hearing about a problem early in its course one can often avoid interruption at a later, less opportune time. The need to make you or a member of your team available to the patient after surgery is dictated largely by the fact that no "postop" rounds are done on patients that have been promptly discharged home.

➥ Call your patients in the evening to see if they are having problems or make it easy for them to reach you if necessary.

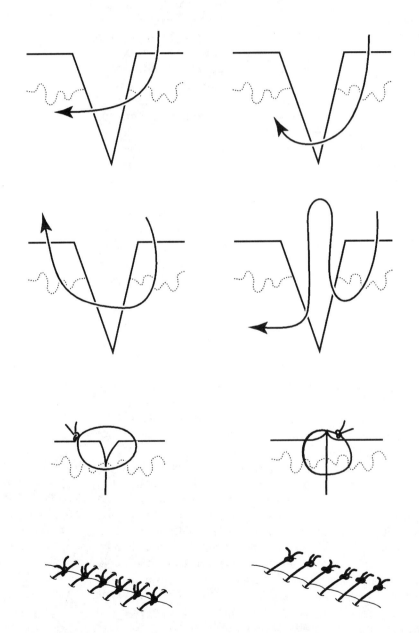

10

Basic Excisional Surgery

PLANNING THE EXCISION

The cornerstone of skin surgery is the elliptical excision. This technique, also known as the fusiform excision, requires the skill and judgment common to almost every other form of advanced skin surgery such as flaps or grafts. The physician who masters the elliptical excision and closure will find it relatively easy to progress to more advanced procedures. They are all variations on the same theme.

Excisional surgery is indicated both for diagnosis and treatment and is *the* procedure by which the skin surgeon demonstrates his or her expertise. Although healing is somewhat dependent on individual patient tendencies, poor technique can almost guarantee a poor scar and excellent technique may often compensate for modest intrinsic healing ability. In excisional surgery, the goal of the physician, aside from removing the offending lesion, is to obtain a scar that is thin and little noticed. Suboptimal scars might be highlighted by their tendency to be red, pigmented, raised, or to cast a shadow. They might be noticeably irregular or wide.

The elliptical excision is valuable when it is necessary to diagnose a lesion in its entirety. For example, when confronted with a pigmented lesion that is suspicious for melanoma, the ideal biopsy approach is to remove complete lesion so that the pathologist may evaluate its full depth. A partial biopsy, such as a punch biopsy, may be confounded by sampling error. An elliptical excision and closure, however, will allow analysis of the whole specimen and

Basic Excisional Surgery

→ To determine the clinical extent of a basal cell cancer after anesthetizing it, curette it. Next, design your excision with 3–5 mm margins.

permit reexcision with margins if indicated. For therapeutic purposes, the elliptical excision is advantageous in the management of nonmelanoma skin cancer, superficial melanoma, and other tumors of the skin.

The process of excisional surgery does not begin when the belly of the scalpel blade strikes the skin. Rather, it is initiated when the surgeon evaluates the lesion to be treated and makes judgments about the anatomic areas at risk, orientation of the scar [Figure 10-1], and the impact on adjacent structures. For example, when evaluating a 5 mm basal cell cancer just inferior to the lateral canthus of the eye, the physician must have an understanding of the thickness of the local skin, the impact of a particular closure on the alignment

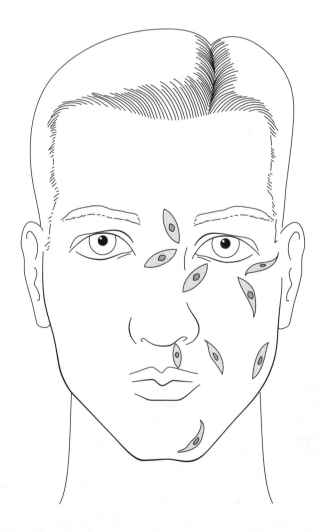

Figure 10-1. Suggested Excision Lines
In order to obtain the best cosmetic result, the scar should be oriented within the lines of facial expression.

150

of the lower lid margin, and the type of suture that would be easiest to place and remove, given the proximity to the eye.

After the surgeon has identified the lesion, discussed with the patient the various options, and reviewed the patient's medical history and contraindications for surgery, the patient is ready for final marking and preparation. When working on the face, it is best to have the patient in a sitting position so that the impact of gravity on natural skin tension lines can be incorporated into the planned excision. Similarly, when planning an excision on the back, especially on the upper shoulder, it is best to have the patient with arms by the side so that there is as natural an anatomic placement of the excisional scar as possible. When operating in the neck area, with the neck turned to one side, the closure may seem particularly tight, but with the patient in the anatomic front forward position, the procedure is facilitated.

MARKING THE LESION

Several options exist for marking the lesion and defining the extent of excision margins. An indelible marker such as a Sharpie is popular with many surgeons as it is convenient, tends not to dry out, and can be reused. A traditional marking technique uses gentian violet dye. In this case, the dye is kept in a small container and the broken end of a cotton tip application is used as a stylus. Although this dye is an excellent marking agent, after cleaning up the tenth spilled vial of gentian violet, one might be persuaded to use a more physician-friendly device. Gentian violet marking pens are available, but they are not predictably sufficiently well inked. The disadvantage of the Sharpie marking pen is that occasionally a tattoo can develop if the marking agent is not completely removed prior to closure.

After the lesion has been identified, it is good to make a dotted outline around its clinical margins. Most cutaneous lesions are circular and one would expect to have a circular pattern outlined. Beyond this, another concentric circle including the margin of normal skin that has been selected is then marked. For a basal cell or squamous cell carcinoma that is clearly defined clinically, a margin of 3–4 mm of normal skin is adequate. For a lentigo maligna, 5 mm of normal skin is indicated, and for a melanoma up to 1 mm in depth, 1 cm margins all around the lesion are currently indicated [Table 10-1].

Once a second concentric circle has been marked in a dotted fashion, if the lesion is on the face it is appropriate to have the patient run through a variety of facial expressions such as grimacing,

Basic Excisional Surgery

TABLE 10-1 Recommended Margins of Excision

Diagnosis	Margins (cm)
Nodular basal cell carcinoma	0.3
Well-circumscribed squamous cell cancer	0.5
Lentigo maligna	0.5
Stage I melanoma (up to 1.0 mm)	1.0

▶ When modifying your design of a wound, use the sharp, broken end of the cotton-tipped applicator and dip in the wound fluid to gently use as a temporary marking agent.

opening the mouth wide, and pursing the lips. This accentuates the relaxed skin tension lines of the face and will help you to determine the direction of the ellipse. The final ellipse should then be marked with the pen. Remember that Christopher Wren did not conceive Westminster Abbey without drawings and you should not proceed with your masterpiece without similarly first casting your design in ink. In fact, the carpenter's adage of "measure twice, cut once" is perhaps more meaningful for facial skin than for Grade 3 Douglas fir.

THE ELLIPSE

The fundamental rule of excisional surgery is that a circular wound must be converted into a fusiform pattern either prior to or during closure, so that when the two sides of the defect are approximated there will be no redundant cones of skin at either end. Proper orientation of the excision is important, but so to is an understanding of how redundant cones of skin, or "dog ears," develop. These would heal as unsightly puckers [Figure 10-2], a phenomenon often worth explaining to the patient.

Special concern arises when the patient presents with a 5 mm lesion—which he or she always believes is smaller than its measured size would suggest—and leaves the office with a 2 cm linear scar. Patients who sew understand the concept of darts that develop when a shirt sleeve is sewn into shirt holes. Similarly, most patients understand that converting a circular wound into a straight line results in redundancies at either end that must be removed and will result in elongation of the scar. Patients are rarely upset about this, but it is important to advise them of the mechanics so that they truly understand why you are doing what you must.

Normally, the vertices of the ellipse are approximately 30 degrees, but they can vary substantially depending on the elasticity

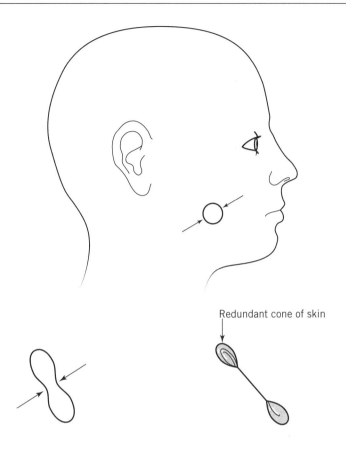

Figure 10-2. Puckers
To minimize the development of redundant cones of skin, also known as "dog ears" or "puckers," it is important to make sure that the ellipse has been designed with adequate length.

of the skin, the location, underlying concavity or convexity, and a need to accommodate other aesthetic goals [Figure 10-3].

ANESTHESIA

Once the lesion has been marked appropriately and the ellipse has been outlined in a dotted fashion, it is time to anesthetize. Often injection in a ring distribution is adequate to obtain anesthesia in the surgical field. It is important to anesthetize beyond the demarcated margins in anticipation of undermining. When the presence of scar presents a concern during a reexcision, additional anesthesia to the base of the wound is necessary. Scar tissue can envelop terminal nerves and inhibit the access of local anesthesia.

Basic Excisional Surgery

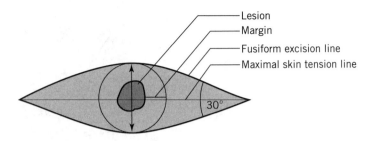

Figure 10-3. Ellipse
The classic design of the ellipse involves a 30-degree angle at either end. However, when the ellipse is being designed over a curvature, either convex or concave, or if skin is especially redundant, the 30-degree angle can be modified.

During blunt undermining and excision of the scarred tissue the patient can feel discomfort. This is best obviated by anesthetizing and waiting 10 or 15 minutes for the anesthetic to take effect. Occasionally it may be easier to perform a nerve block. Although the discomfort from local anesthetic injection is something about which all patients will complain to one degree or another, the anesthetic effect is usually instantaneous and the discomfort is very short-lived. In addition, in areas where one wants to protect underlying structures, infiltration with an abundant amount of anesthesia can distend the tissue and provide a margin of comfort for undermining and excision.

DRAPE AND PREPARATION

Prior to draping and prepping, you and all active staff should don sterile gloves, masks, and appropriate eye protection. Federal guidelines for universal precautions should be followed closely. Once the operative site has been anesthetized, it is necessary to prep the patient with antiseptic [Table 10-2]. The antiseptic should be applied on a gauze 2 × 2, in a circular fashion that spirals from the center outward. Drape either with a precut paper drape or a cloth drape folded at angles so that the whole surgical field is protected. It is also advantageous to place a drape over the patient's eyes so that the bright surgical lights will not be offending.

Drape and Preparation

Do not underestimate the value of talk-esthesia: speak to the patient. Most patients are quite anxious and conversational distraction provides a substantial amount of comfort, often more than chemical compounds. Always tell the patient what you are doing unless the patient explicitly requests not to be told. This occasionally happens, and the patient's request should be honored.

Confirm that all your instruments are in place on the tray, your electrocautery device is handy, suction is available and turned on, lighting is exactly as you want it, and your assistant is in position. Next, prepare the scalpel handle with a scalpel blade, placing the blade into position using the hemostat on the tray. Gently touch the surgical site with the tip of the scalpel and ask the patient if he or she feels anything. The patient will often say: "I feel pressure." Occasionally he or she will say: "It feels sharp." If so, with the tip

➤ Never use Hibiclens near the eyes. pHisoderm is a safe alternative that does not stain the skin like iodine-based preparations.

TABLE 10-2 Antiseptic Agents

Agent	Advantage	Disadvantage
Isopropyl alcohol	Inexpensive Denatures protein including bacterial cell wall	Weak antimicrobial activity Corrosive to instruments Flammable in the setting of cautery Skin irritant
Hexachlorophene (pHisohex)	Strong antigram positive effect	Little effect on gram-negative organisms, fungi Absorbed through skin with potential neurotoxicity in infants Teratogen
pHisoderm*	Broad coverage No absorption Nontoxic	Not irritating to eyes
Chlorhexidine Hibiclens	Broad coverage No absorption Nontoxic Prolonged suppression of bacterial growth	Irritating to eyes and middle ear (keratitis)
Hydrogen peroxide		No significant antiseptic properties Cytotoxic to epidermal cells in culture
Iodoform	Broad spectrum including fungi	Skin irritant Residual color

*Authors' choice

Basic Excisional Surgery

of the local anesthesia needle, try to demarcate the areas where the patient can still feel sensation and extend the anesthesia. Be careful not to perforate the skin, as may be done by eager second-year medical students performing a pin-prick neurology exam.

PROCEDURE

Once you have determined that the patient is adequately anesthetized, apply three-point traction and with the anterior belly of the blade in position over the previously drawn fusiform lines, press down gently and draw in one firm, constant stroke along one side

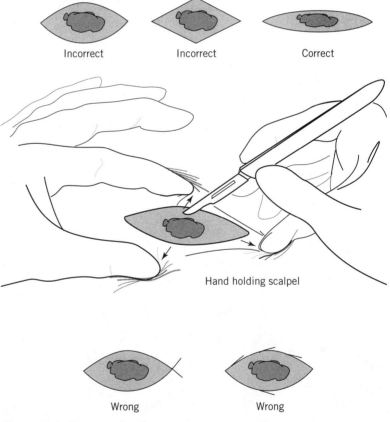

Figure 10-4. Constant Stroke
It is important to incise in a single confident stroke to minimize the risk of a sloppy wound edge.

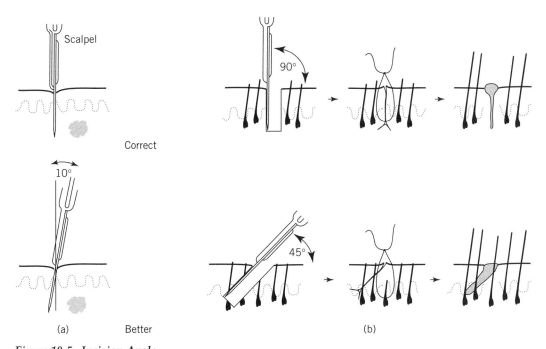

Figure 10-5. Incision Angle
(a) The incision angle should be 10 degrees slightly inward. This is especially true on the back where the bulk of the thick skin can often bulge out and prevent proper apposition. (b) In hair-bearing skin, incision on an angle permits the hair to grow through the scar minimizing its appearance. Modified from Swanson, N. A., 1987 Atlas of Cutaneous Surgery, *Little Brown, Boston.*

of the fusiform ellipse [Figure 10-4]. Do not use jerky, unconfident strokes or you will end up with a jerky, chaotic scar. Once this is done, proceed to the other side. You may encounter a very active blood vessel. If you do, it is certainly acceptable to put the scalpel on the tray, obtain the electrocautery device, and cauterize the affected site. More often than not, you will be able to finish your two preliminary incisions without interruption. As you incise, it is important to anticipate that the two wound edges will, in a short time, be approximated with sutures. Although one normally incises at 90 degrees, there are circumstances when a bevel is indicated (see p. 171). For example, in hair-bearing skin, the incision should be made at approximately 45 degrees which permits the hair to grow through the scar, thus assisting camouflage. In the very thick skin of the back, where a 90-degree incision is likely to yield bulging of the thick dermis and prevent good approximation of the wound, a 10-degree inward incision is advantageous [Figure 10-6].

Basic Excisional Surgery

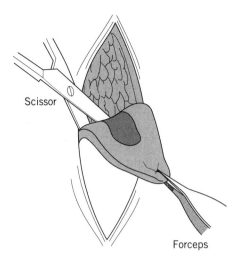

Figure 10-6. Removal of Specimen
Undermine the specimen and lift gently taking care not to crush the specimen edge with the forceps. Use of a hook to elevate the specimen is preferable and avoids the risk of crush artifact.

When the two edges of the wound are approximated, there will be no inhibitory bulging. Ultimately, the goal of the incision, regardless of the location, is to obtain eversion of the wound edges when approximated. After these incisions have been made, take a straight or curved iris scissors and forceps or hook and gently elevate one end of the fusiform ellipse. Insert the scissors through the subcutis in that area and complete the incision through the subcutis along both sides of the specimen. Next, undermine the base of the wound completely and elevate the specimen [Figure 10-6]. Place it onto your tray in an easily identifiable container such as a medicine glass, so that it can be properly removed, marked, and placed in the biopsy specimen bottle.

Hemostasis

➥ If you are going to allow a wound to heal by second intention, compress the edges after cautery to identify additional oozing or vessels that might not be completely sealed.

At this point it is likely that you will have many small oozing vessels in the subcutis and, more likely, at the dermal wound edge. In fact, sites at the wound edge, which correspond anatomically to the papillary dermal blood vessels, are the most frequent bleeders. Often, even when the wound base and the undermined areas are completely dry, patients can develop hematomas from bleeding just at the wound edge itself. It is important, therefore, to identify all bleeding edges and determine whether cautery is indicated.

The use of cautery is considered by some to be a double-edged sword. On the one hand, it is important to minimize bleeding and avoid the postoperative complications related to it. On the other, excessive cautery of tissue is said to delay wound healing. Our extensive experience with electrocautery has not revealed an increased incidence of infection or wound problems. Wound-healing difficulties are more often related to sebaceous skin, therapeutic blood thinners, and diabetes.

Tissue Handling

The goal of minimizing tissue trauma must be pursued at all times. At no time is this more important than when one removes the specimen and begins manipulating the wound edges. Remember that it is the wound edge that will be doing most of the biological work of healing and it is therefore important to treat it with respect if you would like the scar to be something that others would respect. We prefer to use the single-prong skin hook. Occasionally, forceps can be used when the tissue is well-vascularized and even minimal trauma is unlikely to have a sustaining effect.

➥ When working on the face, a disposable hairnet is useful to keep the hair away from the surgical field.

The skin hook should be placed immediately under the wound edge and held at a 90-degree angle [Figure 10-7]. Excessive tension is very often placed on the skin hook or it is held at an acute angle. This is often not very helpful. The greatest visibility is obtained when a skin hook is pulled 90 degrees vertically. A pocket, with the dermis forming the roof and the subcutis the floor, is then available for visualization. It is at this point that we remind students and residents to "visualize and cauterize." It is not reasonable to cauterize blindly as you will have as much chance of effectively cauterizing an offending vessel as you would have of catching pickles blindfolded bobbing in a briny barrel. Better to withstand the sight of a relatively rapid ooze until the opportunity exists to identify the source and cauterize it than to cauterize away blindly in a wet field where the cautery has no practical effect.

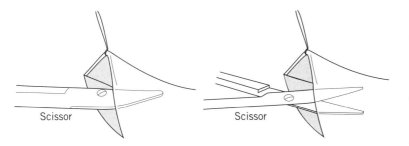

Figure 10-7. Skin Hooks
Skin hooks are an excellent means of manipulating the wound edge in an atraumatic fashion. They should be held at 90 degrees to provide easy visualization of the surgical pocket.

Basic Excisional Surgery

TIPS FOR KEEPING THE WOUND DRY Several tips come to mind with respect to obtaining a dry field. First, wall or Gomco suction is helpful to clear an area that is rapidly filling with blood, as when one encounters an arterial pumper. Second, the most cumbersome challenge to hemostasis occurs with relatively diffuse oozing. Under these circumstances, it is best to take a sponge or gauze and place it in a pocket of tissue with some firm pressure for approximately 10 seconds. The sponge is removed quickly and the bleeder location can be identified. This is really the only way to identify the three or four bleeding sites that are usually all that underlie a relatively large accumulation of blood. Once the sponge has been rapidly removed by recalling the sites that are affected, one can zero in with the electrocautery tip and cauterize before additional blood has accumulated to obscure the view.

Third, an additional helpful device is the cotton-tip applicator. Have 10 or 15 of these on your tray at all times. Your assistant can roll the cotton tip over the affected area while you cauterize behind as a transiently dry bed is created. The cotton-tip applicator is also good for reaching into tight recesses to obtain some tamponade while you attempt to cauterize.

Finally, it will occasionally be necessary to tie off vessels. This usually occurs in the temple area, where branches of the temporal artery are encountered. Normally, however, most vessels are easily cauterized. You should be certain that the vessel you are cauterizing is not so large that it is just temporarily stopped and might later bleed again, especially in patients with elevated blood pressure. The method for tying vessels is demonstrated in Figure 10-8.

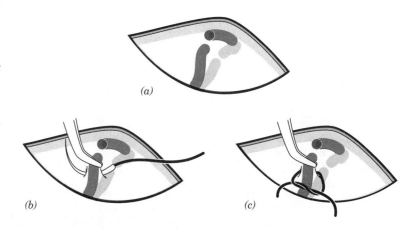

Figure 10-8. Tying Sutures for Bleeders
Ligation of larger vessels such as those that are branches of the temporal artery is often necessary as cautery is insufficient. Place the suture around the vessels and tie. Alternatively, if a blood vessel is actively bleeding, clamp it with a hemostat, slide a suture down along it, tie it, and remove the hemostat when secure.

TABLE 10-3 Suggested Levels of Undermining

Scalp	Below hair follicles or below galea
Forehead	Low subcutaneous tissue—Caution: frontalis muscle
Temple	High subcutaneous tissue—Caution: nerves
Cheeks, chin	High subcutaneous tissue
Lips (mucosa)	Beneath mucosa, above muscle
Nose	Mid or low subcutaneous tissue—above cartilage
Neck	High subcutaneous tissue
Trunk	Any level above muscle fascia
Extremities	Any level above muscle fascia
Hands, feet	Below dermis in areolar tissue

Modified from Bennett, R. G., 1988, Fundamentals of Cutaneous Surgery, Mosby, St. Louis, MO.

Undermining

After the wound bed has been appropriately cauterized, attention must be turned to undermining [Table 10-3]. Undermining is the method by which the adjacent skin is loosened sufficiently to permit approximation of the wound edges with a minimum amount of tension. The amount of undermining that is necessary varies, depending on the location of the defect and the intrinsic elastic qualities of the skin. In elderly patients, where the skin is especially loose, no undermining may be necessary. When not indicated, undermining should not be done because it increases the risk of bleeding. However, in cases where the skin is not sufficiently lax to be approximated without tension, undermining is critical to obtaining a good cosmetic result.

Some suggest that it is necessary to undermine approximately one inch around the excised area to obtain the best possible results. Although this amount may vary, the apices are one region of the ellipse that are always important to undermine. Very often the redundant cones of skin that result from closure of the ellipse will, in time, settle down if the underlying tissue has been loosened. This is analogous to allowing a wrinkle in a bedspread to flatten with time.

Undermining is best performed by trying to minimize trauma to the wound edge. Remember, it is the wound edge that will be approximated and will perform most of the biological work of wound healing. Undermining should always be initiated with the scissors closed. The undermined plane should then be developed by opening the scissor blades. Undermine under direct visualization at as high a level as possible. Be cognizant of important nerves and other structures that are located in your plane of dissection.

➥ When suturing in the scalp, avoid trimming hair. Use a water-soluble lubricant like K-Y Jelly or Surgilube to compact the hair and keep it out of the incision line while tying knots.

Basic Excisional Surgery

➡ When suturing a small wound you may find it difficult to place all the buried sutures. You may find it easier to place the deep sutures and leave them untied. After they are all in place, close the wound by tying the untied knots.

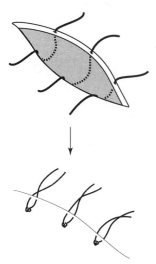

WOUND CLOSURE

Once the lesion has been excised and the wound has been undermined approximately 2 cm in all directions, it is necessary to focus on wound closure. Traditionally, the layered plastic closure consists of a dermal layer of interrupted absorbable sutures and an epidermal layer of nonabsorbable sutures such as Prolene or nylon. The latter are normally removed from 3–10 days postop depending on the location on the body.

Although there are many different approaches, it is often advantageous to close the wound solely with buried sutures and approximate the epidermis with taped closures such as Steri-Strips. With this method, there is less risk of puncture suture marks (fang marks). Furthermore, the patient does not have to return for suture removal and the risk of wound infection is minimized. The advantage to placing epidermal sutures is an improved approximation of the wound edges. It should be stressed that in areas of high tension where the risk of suture marks is greater, closure with deep sutures alone is often sufficient to obtain the best functional and cosmetic result.

Good suturing depends on grasping the needle holder properly [Figure 10-9]. In addition, it permits easy knot tying as demonstrated in Figure 10-10A. There is some debate about the sequence of suture placement. Figure 10-10B shows the range of knots that can be used.

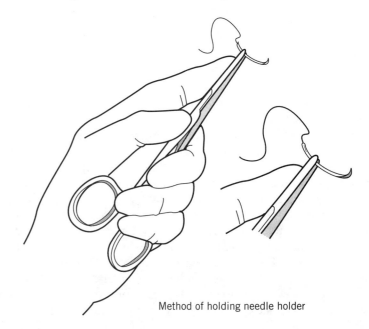

Method of holding needle holder

Figure 10-9. Holding the Needle Holder
The needle holder should be held in a comfortable fashion with the handles placed in the palm of your hand. Your index finger should be placed over the tip of the needle holder so that you can obtain maximal control.

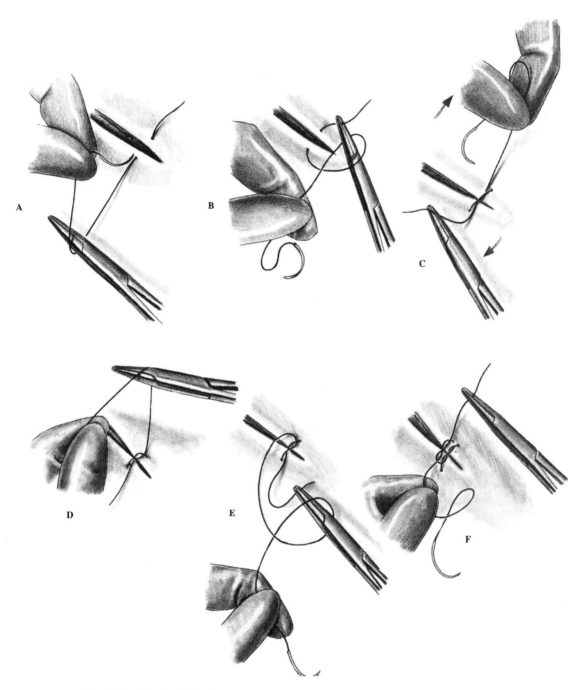

Figure 10-10(A). Tying Surgical Knots
This series demonstrates the proper method for tying surgical knots. The best approach to tying knots is to practice them repeatedly until it becomes possible for you to perform them on a reflex basis. Figures 10-10A and B are reprinted with permission from Bennett, R. G., 1988, Fundamentals of Cutaneous Surgery, *Mosley, St. Louis, MO.*

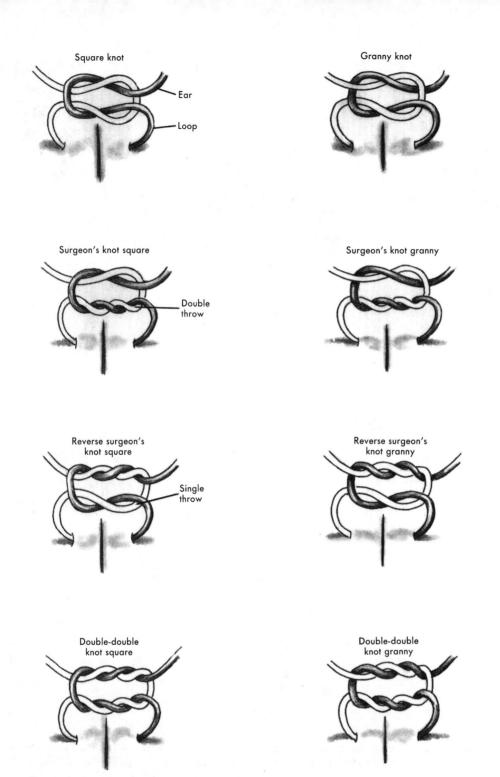

Figure 10-10B.
A variety of surgical knots are demonstrated here. The surgeon's knot square is probably the most versatile.

Wound Closure

It is practical to place the first suture in the middle of the wound and then bisect each half in sequential fashion with additional buried sutures [Figure 10-11]. There are situations where it is best to start at one end and work progressively toward the opposite end of the wound. This is especially true when a wound initially appears to be under tension. Because of the elastic properties of the skin, initial wound tension should not be especially disconcerting. In the course

Initial suture placement

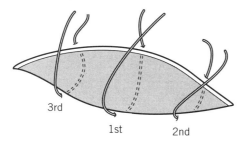

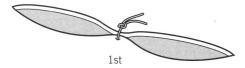

Alternative method

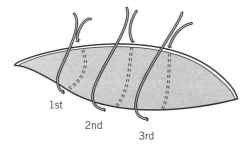

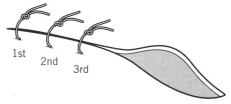

Figure 10-11. Initial Suture Placement
These two approaches to suture placement may be used interchangeably.

Basic Excisional Surgery

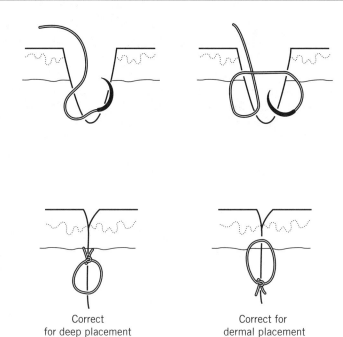

Figure 10-12. Buried Suture
The buried suture is the keystone of the proper surgical closure. It is designed so that the knot lies buried within the depth of the tissue. This helps minimize spitting reactions. The suture must be introduced deep and exit following the arc of the needle. It then enters the opposite side at the same level and passes through the arc of the needle where it comes out to meet its sister on the opposite side. Note that when the buried suture is tied the ends should be pulled perpendicular to the axis rather than parallel to it, which is the case with surface sutures.

of half an hour, one can easily observe resolution of tension due to a unique quality of the integument known as *skin creep*. By initiating closure at one end of the wound and placing sutures every several millimeters so the total tension is distributed evenly over multiple sutures, a wound can often be closed that at first appeared impossible to repair.

The path of the buried suture is demonstrated in Figure 10-12. This step is critical to assure eversion of wound edges.

Figures 10-13(*a*) to (*f*) show the series of steps for suturing a wound.

Undermining not only mobilizes skin for closure but will prevent

Figure 10-13. Suture Series
(a) After excision of the ellipse, the wound can be undermined with blunt scissors. This figure demonstrates the use of a skin hook to minimize wound edge trauma. (b) In preparation for suturing, the wound edge is elevated with forceps or a skin hook. Note how the wound edge must be grasped gently by the forceps to minimize tissue trauma. The needle is placed in the jaws of the needle holder and the needle is pushed through its arc to draw the suture through. In this case a running subcuticular suture is initiated at one vertex of the closure and snaked through the length of the wound within the high dermis. (c) The needle is brought out within the wound and grasped again to be placed through the other side of the wound. Figure 10-13c shows how a simple interrupted suture is placed to secure a running subcuticular suture. The suture is brought through and tied and a single throw is placed. The suture is brought across the wound perpendicular to the axis of the wound itself. Another throw is placed in the knot and the sutures are pulled again in a parallel fashion creating a small loop. Additional throws are placed in the suture and the ends are snipped leaving approximately 1/8 in. tails.

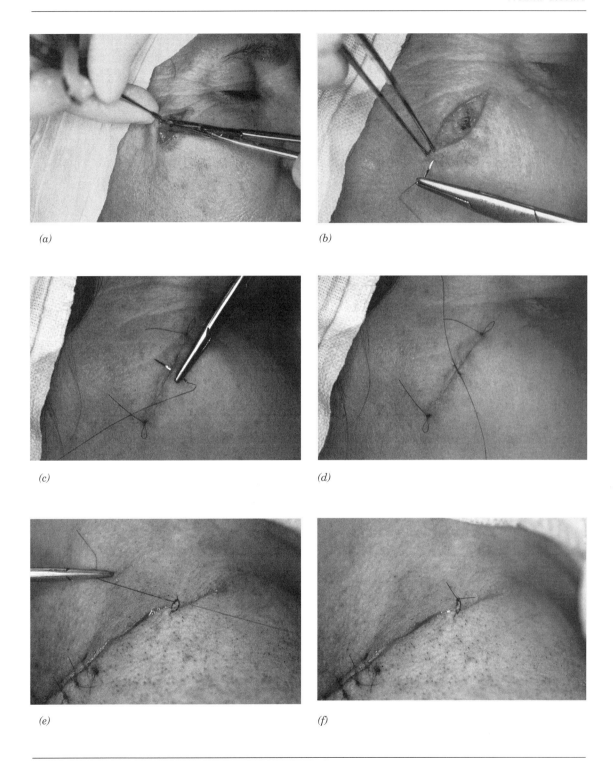

Basic Excisional Surgery

➥ When suturing the ear or other highly vascularized tissue, a running, locking suture is rapid and provides as good hemostasis as interrupted sutures.

buckling of the scar. Buckling and puckering of the scar normally result because a plate of contracting scar tissue develops in the undermined plane. The broader the area of undermining, the less contraction per square centimeter will affect the overlying skin. Levels of undermining are indicated as they vary with locations on the body [Table 10-3]. Vicryl suture or Dexon are useful at most sites. On the scalp and on the extremities, 3-0 Vicryl may be indicated for its added strength, but elsewhere 4-0 Vicryl suffices. In addition, occasionally PDS monofilament is helpful on the back or other high-tension areas because of its superior strength and staying power.

Spitting sutures are a frequent problem with Vicryl sutures and

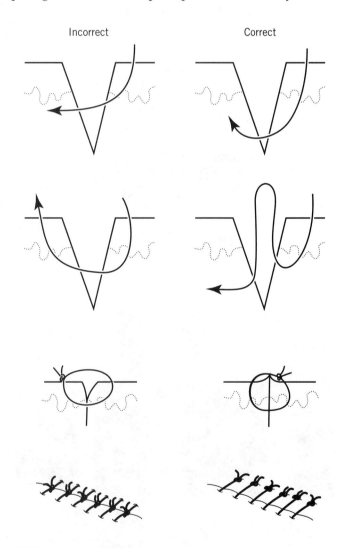

Figure 10-14. Surface Sutures
This suture should be placed approximately 2–3 mm from the wound edge and passed through its natural arc through the dermis and subcutis. It may be brought out between the wound for adjustment. The goal is eversion (right panel). In addition, always slide the final knot to one side of the wound. Knots that lie directly over the incision (left panel) will interfere with healing.

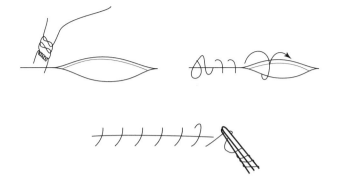

Figure 10-15. Running Sutures
Running sutures are extremely helpful, especially when there is not much tension on the wound. They are simple to place and quick to remove.

all patients should be advised that at approximately 3–4 weeks after surgery they may develop a small pimple at the surgery site. This does not represent a recurrence of the original problem or cancer, but rather the body's attempt at eliminating a Vicryl suture that it has not been able to degrade. For the patient, we analogize this to grass shooting through pavement. It is not uncommon when the patient returns in 3–4 weeks that one or two residual deep sutures will have to be removed, especially over bony areas and where the skin is thin. Selection of sutures will depend on location of the closure, skin type, and type of closure (see Table 10-5).

After the buried sutures have been placed, one can proceed with the epidermal sutures [Figure 10-14]. The simple interrupted suture and the running suture and its variants are the most commonly used [Figures 10-15, 10-16, and 10-17]. Especially helpful are the vertical mattress sutures in areas where the skin naturally inverts [Figure 10-18].

The goal of suture placement, of course, is to have the wound edges everted, so that in time, as the wound spreads slightly (as it inevitably will), the wound edges will lie flat and in closest approximation. The vertical mattress sutures, if removed within 3–6 days, almost never leave suture marks on the face or on areas where the dermis is thicker. They help to flawlessly evert the skin and create a superior result. The buried vertical mattress suture has been discussed in the dermatology literature and in some degree represents

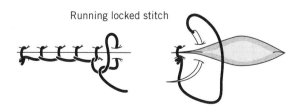

Figure 10-16. Running Locking Sutures
Running locking sutures are beneficial in areas where there is a risk of bleeding. They are especially helpful over the ear, but should not be used where there is a poor blood supply.

Basic Excisional Surgery

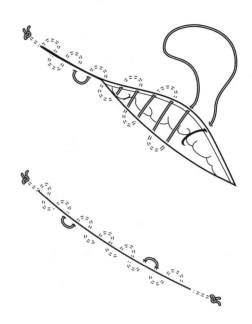

Figure 10-17. Running Subcuticular Sutures
Running subcuticular sutures are practical when there is good approximation with deep sutures. The sutures are snaked through the dermal layer close to the epidermis. It is necessary to remove them cautiously as they may snap in half while extracting at one end. Always bring the suture to the surface every 2–2.5 cm.

an evocation of the epidermal vertical mattress suture that is performed on the surface. This technique and other selective use of suturing options may improve final wound results.

The decision about whether to perform interrupted sutures or running sutures is really one of individual preference [Table 10-4]. On the helix of the ear where blood supply is excellent and tension

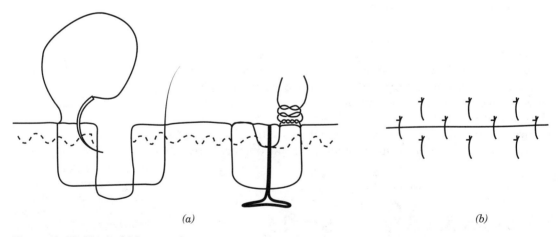

Figure 10-18. Vertical Mattress Suture
This is a very helpful suture in areas of tension. It is excellent for everting wound edges. These sutures should not be left in more than 5 days. (a) Vertical mattress suture. (b) Vertical mattress alternating with simple interrupted sutures.

TABLE 10-4 Running Versus Interrupted Sutures

Factor	Interrupted	Running
Even tension	Yes	No
Hemostasis	Yes	+/−
Selective removal	Yes	No
Speed of placement	No	Yes
Use when no underlying wound tension	Yes	Yes
Eversion control	Yes	No

from cartilage is a concern, the running locking suture is effective. In all other areas where there is good approximation based on the underlying dermal sutures, interrupted or running sutures can be placed. Running sutures are best reserved for situations where approximation of the wound is otherwise excellent and no further refinement is needed with the epidermal sutures.

Simple interrupted sutures are indicated when hematoma is a concern. In this case, one will want to be able to remove one or two sutures to explore the area. If a running suture is placed, the whole closure will have to be untied. In a similar vein, when continued bleeding is a concern it is reasonable to place a wick, either consisting of a Penrose drain or a small length of gauze. This should be placed at the inferior end of the wound where gravity will enhance drainage. The gauze or drain is intended to keep the wound open and will not act as a true channel or conduit. Excessive blood will naturally find the course of least resistance and, after 24 hours, such a wick can be removed. There is no need to place a suture where the wick has been, as this area will close well on its own by second intention over the ensuing week.

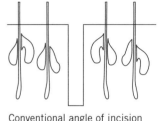

Conventional angle of incision

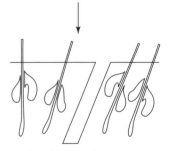

In sebaceous skin use complementary bevels

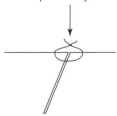

LAZY S REPAIR

Over complex convex surfaces such as the arm, forearm, or lower extremities, a simple linear closure is likely to result in buckling considering there will be up to a 30% shortening of the scar over time. Thus, we design a fusiform ellipse that elongates the scar so that when contraction does occur, buckling will not result. Figure 10-19 demonstrates this technique in detail. Although it appears to result in a longer scar than would ordinarily be anticipated, the final cosmetic result is well worth it. The "S" shape of the design allows for both sufficient elongation and curvilinear alignment of the scar over the convex surface.

➤ When closing wounds on very sebaceous skin, bevel one edge in and the opposite edge out. The two sides of the wound will then come together like a shirt inside pants and yield a superior result without the typical delling that can otherwise develop.

Figure 10-19. Lazy S Excision
The Lazy S excision is indicated when closing lesions over convex surfaces. It elongates the actual length of the scar so that the natural scar contraction that occurs in time will not result in buckling. Reprinted with permission from Swanson, N. A., 1988, *Atlas of Cutaneous Surgery,* Little Brown, Boston.

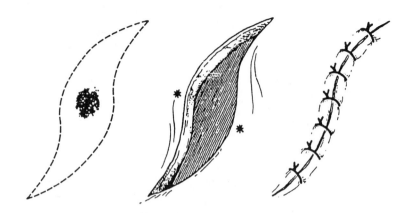

M-plasty

Often, when a linear incision is performed, the "dog ear," or extension of the ellipse, can impinge on important areas such as the lateral canthus of the eye or the vermillion border of the lip. To minimize the extension of the nonpathologic end of the repair into these important regions, a foreshortening technique referred to as M-plasty can be performed. In essence, rather than extend the ellipse completely to include the 30-degree angle at the end, an "M" pattern is created at approximately one-quarter of the way down the ellipse. Figure 10-20 demonstrates this technique in sequence. It is simply an alternative method for removing the dog ear which is described in Figure 10-21. A tip stitch is very helpful in completing the M-plasty [Figure 10-22].

Dog Ears

It is extremely common when performing an ellipse to obtain redundant cones of skin at either end of the wound. These "darts" result because of the conversion of a circular defect into a linear repair. There are several different approaches to repair "dog ears." The purpose of removing the excess tissue is to optimize the cosmetic result. Although in older patients such redundancies may well fall out in time, in younger patients they will not, especially in sebaceous skin and they can be the source of much cosmetic concern.

After the repair has been performed and there is a redundancy at one or both ends, the residual skin may be excised: (1) as an additional small ellipse; (2) by extending the defect; or (3) by an incision made by lifting up the dog ear with a skin hook and draping the excess tissue over the side of the wound [Figure 10-21]. Another incision is made to excise the excess tissue such that the line is

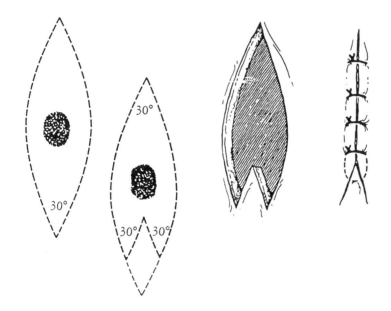

Figure 10-20. M-plasty
M-plasty permits foreshortening of the scar to avoid extension into significant cosmetic areas such as the eyebrow, lip, and eyelid area. Reprinted with permission from Swanson, N. A., 1987, Atlas of Cutaneous Surgery, Little Brown, Boston.

directly contiguous with the previous excision line. Occasionally, it may be advantageous to remove dog ears along the length of the wound. When removing the dog ear, the "hockey stick technique" often results in a curvilinear line that is usually superior to the "T" or "M" revision of a dog ear.

After the sutures have been placed, it is important to compress the wound gently and determine whether there is any residual bleeding. Compression of the surgical site for approximately 5 minutes after the surgery minimizes postoperative swelling. In addition, if there is some minimal wound edge bleeding, this too can be controlled with pressure for 5 minutes. This is a good opportunity to demonstrate to the patient how he or she should apply pressure at home if bleeding should develop. Patients invariably do not apply enough pressure or vastly underestimate 5 minutes. That is why we always instruct patients to apply pressure for 5–10 minutes *by the clock.*

➥ Although it is important to cut sutures with short tails so they do not become trapped in the healing wound, when cutting sutures on the scalp, leave the tails a bit longer so they can be easily found at the time of removal.

Dressing

After adequate pressure has been applied, we routinely bandage the site with a layer of Polysporin or petrolatum ointment followed by a nonstick dressing such as Telfa, a few gauze pads for a pressure effect, and tape [Figure 10-23]. It is best to eschew Neosporin because of the risk of allergic reactions. In addition, recent data suggests that antibiotic ointment is no better at protecting against infection than petrolatum or other similar nonantibacterial agents. Patients that are

Basic Excisional Surgery

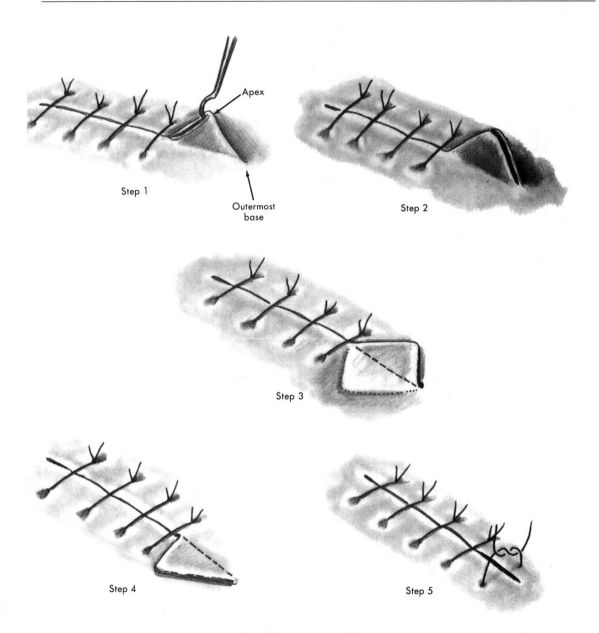

Figure 10-21. Dog-Ear Techniques
Redundant cones of skin or "dog ears" can be removed in several ways. Reprinted with permission from Bennett, R. G., 1988, Fundamentals of Cutaneous Surgery, Mosby, St. Louis, MO.

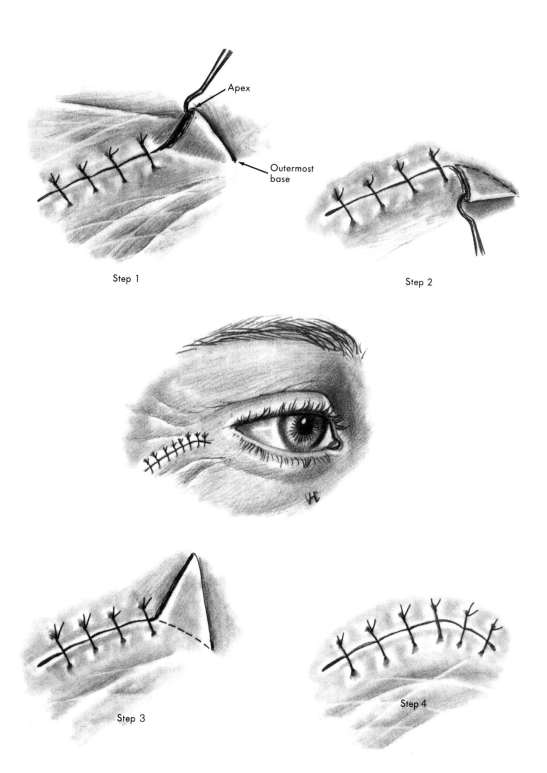

Step 1

Step 2

Step 3

Step 4

Basic Excisional Surgery

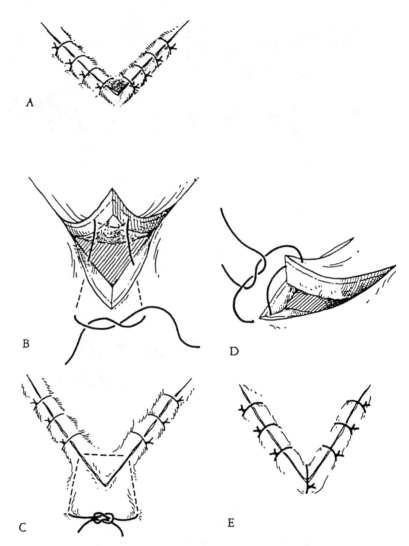

Figure 10-22. Tip Stitch
The tip stitch allows excellent apposition of the wound edges when an M-plasty is performed. Reprinted with permission from Swanson, N. A., 1987, Atlas of Cutaneous Surgery, Little Brown, Boston.

allergic or sensitive to adhesive are treated with Scanpore hypoallergenic tape. Alternatively, we much prefer to use an elasticized flesh-colored tape called Hy-Tape. It allows a great deal of pressure to be applied in the first 24 hours and has zinc oxide in its adhesive, which seems to be gentle on most skin types.

This pressure dressing can be removed at 24 hours and replaced with a smaller gauze bandage. We advise patients not to place the gauze itself directly over the wound as fibers can easily get trapped in the wound edge, become matted, and delay healing [Table 10-6]. Similarly, when cutting sutures, it is important to cut the tail short enough that it does not get embedded in the wound and inhibit

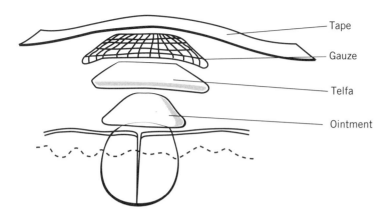

Figure 10-23. Bandage
The bandage that is placed following surgery should be simple and easy for the patient to apply. It must protect the wound from air exposure. This multiple-layer technique involving ointment, Telfa, gauze, and tape permits pressure in the first 24 hours as well. Modified from Bennett, R. G., 1988, Fundamentals of Cutaneous Surgery, *Mosby, St. Louis, MO.*

healing. Sutures can be removed at times indicated in Table 10-7. Proper technique should be used [Figure 10-24].

It is important to note that some surgeons do not use any wound covering during the healing period. We believe the techniques described here are preferable, especially as most patients choose to cover their new wound for cosmetic reasons until sutures are removed.

Specialty Sutures

When performing surgery on the eyelids it is often preferable not to have to remove sutures because of the very fine skin. In this case, 7-0 Vicryl, an expensive but useful suture, is an excellent surface wound closure material. It can be left in place to dissolve on its own, yet provides very good wound-closing strength. It is less reactive than the traditional gut-based sutures.

➥ Use blue sutures in the scalp rather than black ones. They will be easier to identify when it is time to remove them.

Suture Removal

Although a cause of permanent track marks is excessive tension on the sutures, sutures should be removed promptly to avoid epithelial tracts from developing (Table 10-7). If the patient is not able to return for suture removal, but superficial sutures are desired, it is possible to use fast-absorbing chromic sutures in a running fashion and then

TABLE 10-5 Suture Selection

	Buried	Epidermal
Face	4-0, 5-0 vicnyl	5-0, 6-0 prolene
Trunk	3-0, 4-0 vicnyl	4-0, 5-0 prolene
Extremities	3-0, 4-0 vicnyl	3-0, 4-0 nylon 4-0 prolene

Basic Excisional Surgery

TABLE 10-6 Dressing Options

Closure		Dressing Sequence	Comment
None:			
Heal by second intention	1	Polysporin × 1 week and Telfa	Minimal oozing; risk of allergic reaction to Polysporin if prolonged use
		Petrolatum and Telfa until healed	
	2	Silver sulfadiazine × 7-10 days and Telfa	Stimulates granulation tissue; risk of excess granulation from SSD
		Petrolatum and Telfa until healed	
	3	Duoderm; change every two days	Collection of wound fluid; must drain daily; may have to change more frequently
		Switch to petrolatum and Telfa when granulation is maximal	Avoid hypergranulation
Layered Closure: dermal and epidermal sutures	1	Polysporin or petrolatum with telfa until sutures out; Steri-Strips and Mastisol for three days	Clean wound daily with tap water
	2	Tegaderm only until sutures out	Small amount of serous material will collect
dermal sutures only	1	Mastisol, Steri-Strips, and Tegaderm	Very convenient; no wound care required until bandage removed; risk of maceration
	2	Mastisol and Steri-Strips	Minimal care

Note: In all bandage options, a pressure dressing consisting of gauze and elasticized tape is placed for the first 24 hours and then removed by the patient.

TABLE 10-7 Suture Removal

	Days: Minimum	Days: Maximum
Face	3	6
Ears	7	10
Trunk	5	10
Extremities	5	10

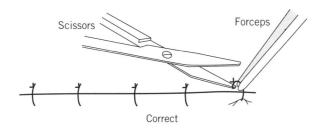

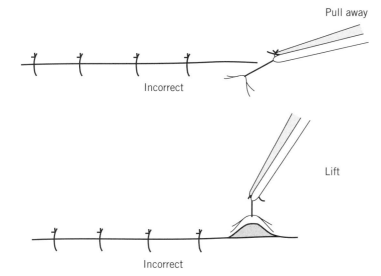

Figure 10-24. Suture Removal
Sutures should be snipped and pulled to the opposite side of the wound to minimize possible unintended dehiscence (top panel). Pulling the suture away from the wound or lifting it may cause the wound edge to separate.

cover the wound with Steri-Strips. Instruct the patient to remove the Steri-Strips in 5 days, the point at which most of the suture has begun to dissolve. The strips will remove any residual gut fragments. Patients react more to gut than to other types of sutures, but if they are removed quickly, such complications can be minimized. The reaction normally presents as swelling, redness, and itching along the repair (see p. 202).

Suture Allergy

There is an occasional patient who is truly allergic to Vicryl sutures. This should be marked clearly on his or her chart and Vicryl should not be used. It is important, however, to elicit a clear history of allergy consisting of persistent redness, bumps, and even pain. Most patients may confuse a spitting suture with an allergic reaction. PDS is an excellent alternative in this situation.

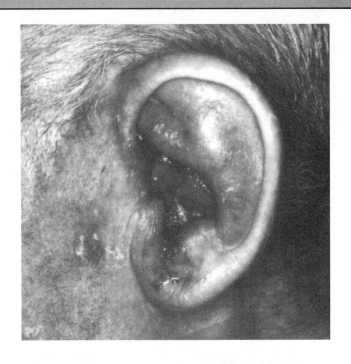
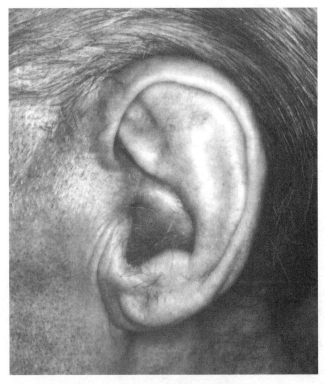

11

Surgical Complications

Surgical complications are unavoidable. If you perform skin surgery and do not experience complications, you are probably not doing enough procedures. No matter how skilled the surgeon or compliant the patient, adverse and undesirable outcomes will occur. Knowledge of these potential complications and the preventative measures that can be taken will smooth the rocky road of suboptimal results. One important preparative step is informed consent. Both patients and physicians must realize that all surgical procedures, no matter how simple, carry adverse outcome risks. The most common complications and their management are reviewed here. It is important to understand that the four most common complications, or terrible tetrad, can tumble like a set of dominos. Bleeding can lead to hematoma, which can cause infection. This in turn can cause necrosis which may be followed by dehiscence [Figure 11-1].

BLEEDING

Bleeding problems are the most commonly encountered surgical complications in the office surgery setting. Profuse or persistent intraoperative bleeding is of concern to the surgeon, and postoperative bleeding can provoke anxiety and stress in the patient. Often, bleeding problems can be prevented through careful attention to preoperative evaluation and preparation. Intraoperative bleeding

Surgical Complications

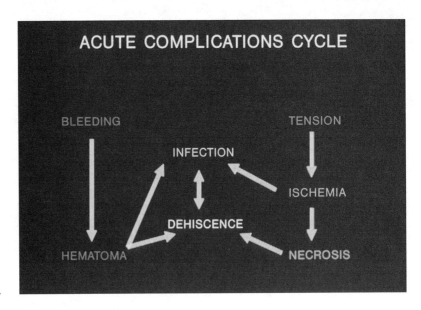

Figure 11-1. Complications Complications in skin surgery can develop as a chain reaction.

can be managed in a temporizing fashion until a dry field is obtained, and postoperative hemorrhage is usually prevented by careful attention to hemostasis.

Causes

MEDICATIONS. Most bleeding complications are related to medications, especially aspirin-containing compounds. Patients may be unaware that the over-the-counter remedy they are using may contain a salicylate. Nonsteroidal anti-inflammatory drugs (NSAIDs) also will inhibit coagulation. Both classes of drugs interfere with platelet function. Platelets normally block the cyclo-oxygenase pathway, leading to platelet aggregation and the formation of thrombus. Aspirin blocks this pathway for the lifespan of the platelet (6–10 days). NSAIDs block the same enzyme but not as severely, and the reversible effect resolves within 3 hours. Patient should stop taking aspirin or NSAIDs at least 1 week prior to surgery and for 5–7 days after surgery. Acetaminophen is an excellent substitute because it does not interfere with coagulation. Patients should be given a complete list with all aspirin- and NSAID-containing compounds to avoid prior to surgery.

➥ As you attempt to obtain hemostasis, especially after undermining, remember to "visualize and cauterize." Your Hyfrecator will not work effectively in a wet field.

Warfarin (Coumadin) is now very commonly used for both cardiac disease and stroke. As the population ages, it is likely that Coumadin will become even more ubiquitous. When feasible, Coumadin should be stopped, but only under the direction and supervision of the patient's primary-care physician or cardiologist. The medication should be discontinued 2 days prior to surgery and reinstituted 1 day after surgery. At times, the risk of stopping the Coumadin is greater than the risk of intraoperative and postoperative bleeding. In general, intraoperative bleeding from aspirin is far more prevalent than from Coumadin. Some dermatologists do not even discontinue the Coumadin if the procedure is not especially complex. Meticulous care should be taken during surgery to control intraoperative bleeding, remembering that the field may be deceptively dry if epinephrine has been used. In the unusual instance of persistent bleeding with Coumadin, parenteral vitamin K or fresh frozen plasma can be administered to instantly reverse its effects.

INCOMPLETE INTRAOPERATIVE HEMOSTASIS. Complete control of bleeding during surgery is critical to prevent postoperative hemorrhage. Intraoperative hemostasis should be approached in a systematic manner. The key to effective hemostasis is good equipment: adequate overhead lighting, suction apparatus, skin hooks to explore under skin edges, cotton-tipped applicators to tamponade areas of bleeding and wick away fluid to create a dry field, and proper electrosurgical equipment. Two hands are never enough to achieve good hemostasis, so a well-trained assistant must be present. Underlying all the technical issues of hemostasis is a golden principle identified by Dr. Leffell as "visualize, then cauterize."

Cautery can be effected in many ways. The popular monopolar Hyfrecator is excellent for control of small bleeding vessels. The sharp-tipped, active electrode can be applied directly to the vessel or bleeding area where it works best in a dry field. Blood dissipates heat, so be aware of excessive thermal injury to obtain a limited amount of hemostasis. Rolling cotton-tipped applicators over the bleeding area will help visualize pin-point bleeding. If blood flow is brisk, then a suction apparatus will usually be necessary to identify the source of the bleeding. Often, once a small pumping vessel is identified and cauterized or ligated, further field visualization will no longer be impaired.

➡ While the plume of electrocautery has never been proven to be dangerous, it is offensive. Hold the plastic tip of your Gomco or other suction device close to the cautery tip. It will keep the field smoke free and the smell away from the patient.

Electrocoagulation should not be excessive ("coagulate but moderate") because it will leave necrotic tissue, which may dispose to increased inflammation, slower healing, and potentially more scarring. The goal of intraoperative hemostasis is to stop bleeding with minimal char and necrosis. Bipolar coagulation (e.g., Bovie) uses a lower voltage and higher frequency to generate less heat and potentially less tissue damage. To achieve this, the patient is grounded with a metal plate, and if bipolar forceps are used, an

Surgical Complications

electric arc across the forcep tips will limit coagulation to the vessel between the forcep tips. Larger bleeding vessels must be clamped and suture ligated to avoid postoperative bleeding.

In hypertensives, or with vessels that do not seal immediately with electrocautery, assume there is risk of clot dislodgment and postoperative bleeding, in which case the safest approach is to tie off the vessel. An absorbable suture (chromic, Dexon, Vicryl, Monocryl) should be used to properly ligate the vessel. If intraoperative bleeding is persistent, despite ongoing electrocoagulation and pressure, consider placing a drain at the surgical site [Figure 11-2A]. A fenestrated ¼ in. Penrose or gauze wick (Nugauze) can be placed in the dead space of the wound to help drain away blood and serosanguinous fluid. This helps to avoid a hematoma at the wound site. The drain should be removed in 24 hours because it can serve as a nidus of infection. The patient should be placed on antibiotics.

ENDOGENOUS BLEEDING. At times bleeding complications may develop because the patient has an acquired or genetic bleeding diathesis. This can usually be identified at the preoperative consultation visit. The patient should be questioned about easy bruisability, prolonged bleeding after minor cuts or dental work, unexplained nosebleeds, and family history of bleeding problems. If there is any suspicion of an acquired or hereditary bleeding coagulopathy, the patient should have screening laboratory blood work, including complete blood count (CBC), platelet count and morphology, bleed-

Figure 11-2. Drain to Prevent Hematoma
(a) A penrose drain can be fenestrated and sutured into the wound to permit drainage of blood if there is risk of hematoma. (b) A piece of Nugauze is placed to serve as a drain in a patient who had significant bleeding during surgery. This prevented the collection of blood. Usually the drain can be removed the day after surgery and the wound will close completely.

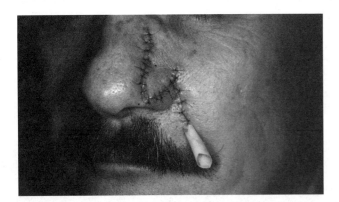

(a)

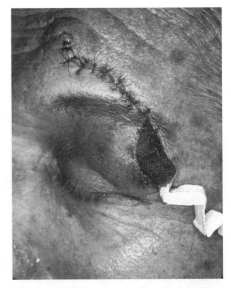

(b)

ing time, prothrombin time (PT), and partial thromboplastin time (PTT). In the vast majority of patients undergoing outpatient cutaneous surgical procedures, these screening laboratory tests are usually not necessary. Laboratory tests do not supplant a complete and thorough history.

Lack of compliance may sometimes dispose patients to bleeding problems. The patient may be told to avoid alcohol due to the vasodilatory effects, but will go home and have several drinks. Likewise, the postoperative patient is instructed to rest and is given explicit instructions about activity. Yet patients may be overzealous with their activity and bleeding can occur. It is important to be very specific about postoperative activity restrictions and how long they must be observed.

Dietary restrictions are especially germane if the surgical wound can be affected by muscles of mastication. The postoperative instruction sheet should detail what the patient should do in case of bleeding. Most bleeding can be controlled with adequate pressure (15–20 minutes) as long as the patient and family have been properly informed and educated. Emphasize that it is 10–20 minutes "by the clock" because there is a tendency to fatigue easily after only a few minutes of holding pressure and then to check the wound to see if it is still bleeding.

> Ice packs are often useful after surgery to control local pain and swelling. However, they may be heavy, and when they melt they become messy. As an alternative, recommend a bag of frozen peas or corn, which is light and can conform to the wound shape.

Management of Bleeding

Bleeding can occur in three settings: (1) acutely during the surgical procedure; (2) during the early postoperative period (2–24 hours postop); or (3) during the late postoperative period (>24 hours). Management guidelines are as follows.

INTRAOPERATIVE BLEEDING. Most bleeding can be controlled with electrocoagulation or suture ligation. If the problem is excessive oozing due to aspirin use, firm pressure may be required for 10–20 minutes. For a wound that will be left open to granulate, an absorbable gelatin sponge can be used. Gelfoam is a sterile, nonantigenic surgical sponge made from animal skin gelatin. It is porous and absorbs many times its weight in blood and fluid. Hemostasis is probably caused by concentration of clotting factors in the sponge itself. Gelfoam is conveniently cut to fit the wound bed and will be slowly absorbed over 4 weeks.

Oxidized cellulose (Oxycel, Surgistat) can also be used for open wounds. This absorbable material is made from cellulose that has been oxidized, so it is soluble and absorbable after tissue implantation. It is available as a gauze pad or knitted fabric strip and is most helpful to control oozing from a broad surface.

Bovine collagen is available in sponge form as well (Instat), or as a loose, fluffy material (Avitene). It produces hemostasis by providing a surface to which platelets can adhere, leading to clot formation. Thrombin (Thrombostat) is a physiologic hemostatic agent that activates fibrinogen to form a fibrin clot. The freeze-dried powder can be reconstituted into a solution and sprayed by syringe onto the wound or bleeding site. Its major drawbacks are expense and the theoretical possibility of intravascular clotting if it enters a larger blood vessel.

Epinephrine in the local anesthetic solution is very helpful to control intraoperative bleeding. The major disadvantage is delayed bleeding after the vasoconstrictive effect has dissipated. Small vessels may completely vasoconstrict, but as the epinephrine effect fades, the vessels will vasodilate to their normal size and begin to bleed. Unfortunately, this usually occurs 2–3 hours after the procedure when the patient has already returned home.

Early Postoperative Bleeding. Most bleeding occurs within the first 6 hours after surgery. Blood may ooze through the suture line and soak the dressing or it may collect under the suture line in the wound dead space and cause an expansile hematoma. The hematoma is heralded by swelling, discomfort, and pain. Early on, the hematoma is a gel-like mass and should be promptly removed. If the hematoma is small, it can be expressed through a small opening in the suture line or aspirated, but typically the sutures will need to be removed completely to remove the hematoma and identify the bleeding source. At times, a small arterial "pumper" will be noted. More commonly, there is simply diffuse oozing, especially if a muscle has been cut or exposed. Bleeding vessels may be found deeply or at the distal extent of the undermined wound.

After the hematoma is removed, the wound should be irrigated with sterile saline and the bleeding should be stopped completely. A drain may be placed and antibiotics should be initiated to minimize infection risk after this extensive tissue trauma. The wound, if on the face, may be safely resutured in the first 24 hours.

Late Postoperative Bleeding. At times, if the hematoma is smaller or develops insidiously, the patient may not detect or report it. The hematoma may be noted initially at suture removal 5–7 days after surgery. If there is no evidence of wound tension or compromise of normal healing, the hematoma can be left alone and allowed to resolve slowly. Between the 7th and 14th postoperative days, the hematoma will actually liquify and can often successfully be aspirated with an 18 gauge needle [Figure 11-3]. If the hematoma is causing tissue necrosis or wound dehiscence, the wound should be

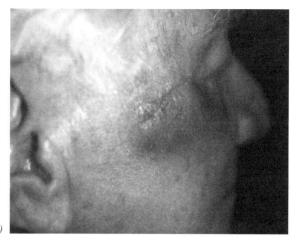

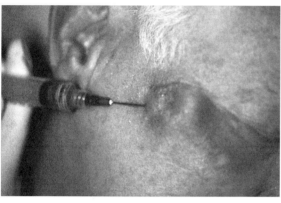
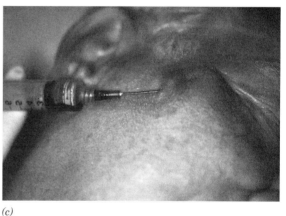

Figure 11-3. Management of Hematoma
(a) This hematoma was first noted 4 days after surgery and the patient became concerned because of the increasing mass. (b) An 18-gauge needle is inserted into the hematoma without local anesthesia. (c) The plunger is withdrawn and old blood is aspirated.

opened and the hematoma evacuated. At 1 week, the wound should probably be left to heal secondarily and not be resutured. The patient will need to be seen on a frequent basis and given reassurance about the healing process.

Prevention of Bleeding

Certain steps can be taken to minimize the risk of bleeding and hematoma.

1. Complete preoperative evaluation and identification of patients at risk is important, including those taking offending medications and those with inherited or acquired bleeding dyscrasias.

2. Stop aspirin, salicylate-containing compounds, and nonsteroidal2anti-inflammatory drugs 1 week prior to surgery. Stop Coumadin 2 days prior to surgery after first checking with the patient's primary-care physician. Do not restart these medications for at least 2–7 days postoperatively.

3. No alcohol is allowed for 48 hours postoperatively.

4. Limit activity appropriate to the size, location, and complexity of the surgical procedure.

5. Give patients detailed wound-care instructions, including directions on how to remove the bandage, how to apply a clean dressing, and how to apply pressure as needed. Patients should be educated about the difference between ecchymosis and bleeding complications. Ecchymosis represents diffusion of blood along dissection planes or natural tissue planes. Final collection may be at dependent sites [Figure 11-4]. For example, the patient should be

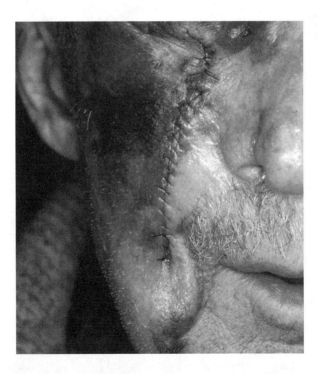

Figure 11-4. Ecchymosis
Ecchymosis can be quite impressive, especially in elderly patients with thin skin. It is important to advise patients that ecchymosis will be subject to gravity and that any surgery on the face may result in ecchymosis down the neck. It usually resolves in one to two weeks.

warned that surgery around the eye (even on the upper forehead) may result in swollen black and blue eyes. Surgery on the cheek may result in bruising in the lower neck area. Ecchymosis alone is benign and resolves in 1–2 weeks.

6. Adequate pressure dressings should be applied for the initial 24–48 hours after surgery. The value of a good pressure dressing cannot be overemphasized. Pressure dressings are extremely valuable in vascular areas such as the scalp or nose. A pressure dressing consists of a bulky, loose gauze, gauze pads, or cotton balls firmly taped into place over a nonstick dressing. Additional pressure can be achieved with elastic bandages, elasticized tape, and tubular gauze. Nursing personnel need to learn the fine art of pressure dressings.

It is wise to see patients who have had significant intraoperative bleeding for an initial wound check and dressing change in 24 hours. All patients should be called at home within the first 24 hours to make sure they are doing well. Careful questioning over the telephone can often highlight specific problems.

INFECTION

Fortunately, wound infections from office-based skin surgery are infrequent (1–3%). When wound infection does occur, however, it can be devastating in terms of prolonged healing time and final cosmetic outcome. Infections can range in severity from moderate erythema and swelling, to purulent abscess formation and systemic infection [Figure 11-5].

A wound infection exists when pathogenic bacteria contaminating the wound overcome local tissue defenses and cause an inflammatory host response. A mild wound infection may be difficult to distinguish from a normally healing wound (which typically will show an element of erythema, swelling, and tenderness secondary to the surgical procedure, trauma, and placement of suture material). Most wound infections will begin between postoperative days 4 and 8, when normal postincisional discomfort and swelling begin to resolve. Clinically, a wound infection will show moderate to marked erythema, edema, warmth, tenderness, and sometimes purulent drainage [Figure 11-6].

A soft-tissue abscess can develop under the suture line. As the infection worsens, so do the signs and symptoms. Lymphatic streak-

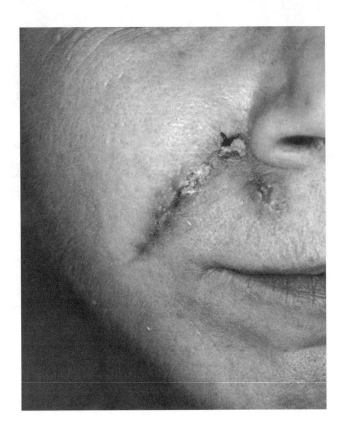

Figure 11-5. Staphylococcal Wound Infection
This situation is relatively rare but can occur, especially if an individual in the operative field, or the patient, happened to be a nasal staph carrier. The infection should be treated with antibiotics. If there is evidence of abscess, the sutures should be opened and drainage should be performed.

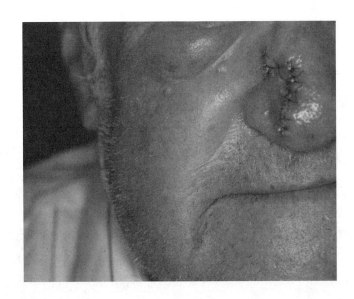

Figure 11-6. Cellulitus
Cellulitis can occur as a result of skin surgery. In this case it developed in spite of antibiotic coverage in a patient who was immune suppressed as a result of lymphoma.

ing, lymphadenopathy, fever, chills, and an elevated white blood cell count suggest systemic infection. Infections, usually controlled without great difficulty with antibiotics, may result in delayed wound healing, possible wound dehiscence, and poor cosmetic outcome.

Infection rates vary based on a number of factors including complexity of the surgical procedure, degree of wound contamination, operative technique, and host factors.

Patient (Host) Factors

The patient's general medical status will affect both wound healing and the risk of infection. Table 11-1 outlines patient risk factors for increased susceptibility to infection.

Patients with underlying systemic medical problems such as diabetes, hepatic and/or renal disease, and myeloproliferative disorders are at obvious risk. Patients in poor physical shape due to obesity, cigarette smoking, malnutrition, and alcohol abuse have increased problems with infection. Any cause of immunosuppression, especially drugs (prednisone, azathioprine, cyclophosphamide, methotrexate, cyclosporine), AIDS, and underlying systemic malignancies, will increase infections. As patients age, their risk of infection increases. Finally, patients who are nasal carriers of *Staphylococcus aureus* will have more problems with postoperative wound infections than others.

TABLE 11-1 Host Factors for Wound Infection

1. Diabetes
2. Liver or kidney disease
3. Malnutrition
4. Alcohol abuse
5. Cigarette smoking
6. Immunosuppression
7. Increasing age
8. Obesity
9. Myeloproliferative disorders
10. *Staphylococcus aureus* carrier

Operative Technique

The best way to prevent wound infection is to practice good technique. Crushed tissue heals poorly, so all good technique begins with gentle handling of tissue. Proper use of skin hooks and toothed forceps minimizes crush injury to skin edges. Excessive tension on the wound edge should be avoided. If closed under tension or with sutures tied too tightly, tissue ischemia and infection may occur. Occasionally, even though a linear closure can be done, a flap may better minimize tension and thus reduce the risk of infection. Poor control of bleeding, especially with hematoma formation, will provide a potential nidus for infection. The hematoma is best thought of as a "Petri dish" for pathogenic skin bacteria. Prolonged operation (greater than 3 hours) will also increase the risk of infection. The extent of excision and complexity of the operation are directly correlated with the risk of wound infection.

Strict adherence to aseptic technique will, of course, decrease the degree of wound contamination. Sources of wound contamination include the patient, operating room personnel, surgical equipment, and the ambient air. Following sterile techniques as closely as possible will minimize contamination and the risk of infection although, of course, it will not eliminate it. Thorough handwashing by every member of the surgical team, preoperative skin prep with chlorhexidine or Betadine, proper instrument sterilization, and use of masks, gowns, and sterile gloves are all aspects of proper sterile technique. The operative site on the patient should be isolated by sterile drapes and towels. Personnel traffic in the room should be limited. Realistically, most office-based procedures will result in minor breaks in aseptic technique and will fall into the clean-contaminated category but striving to minimize infection should be the goal of your office surgery suite routine.

Local Wound Factors

Certain anatomic locations are more susceptible to cutaneous infections, including the perineum, axillae, and lower extremities. Overall, skin surgery of the head and neck does quite well due to excellent vascularity, but the perinasal location can be at increased risk due to potential Staphylococcal colonization of the nose. Previously irradiated tissue has poor vascularity and is at increased risk for infection and poor wound healing. Exposed cartilage, especially in the ear region, is prone to infection, sometimes with *Pseudomonas* [Figure 11-7a and b]. For this reason, acetic acid soaks are recommended to clean the exposed cartilage area postoperatively. Inflammation of

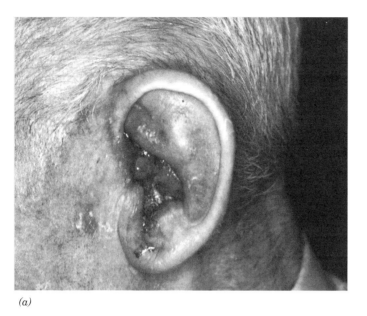 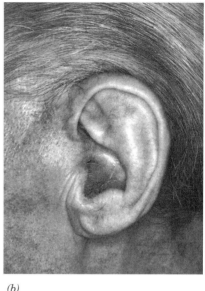

(a)   (b)

Figure 11-7. Pseudomonas Infection
(a) Pseudomonas infection of the ear can result in malignant otitis externa. For this reason, all patients that have ear surgery, especially with exposed cartilage, are placed on ciprofloxacin. (b) Same patient after treatment with ciprofloxacin.

the operative site (inflamed cyst, eroded tumors, or skin ulcerations) will increase infection risk. An infection distant from the surgical site will also increase the potential for wound infection.

Treatment

If there is drainage, a Gram stain and culture and sensitivity should be done. Many times the wound will be red and inflamed but without a pustular exudate. Most wound infections are due to *Staphylococcus aureus*. The best empiric antibiotic treatment includes a penicillinase-resistant penicillin or erythromycin (unless the infection was acquired in the hospital setting). A broad-spectrum cephalosporin will add additional coverage against some Gram-negative organisms. Pseudomonas infections of the ear should be treated with ciprofloxacin.

In most instances, sutures will need to be removed if there is an infection. Sutures may potentiate an infection by interfering with normal host defenses. If an abscess is apparent, it must be drained and the area should be irrigated. Iodoform gauze strips should be inserted into the wound daily until drainage has stopped and second-intention healing can proceed. If necessary, scar revision can be performed several months after healing is complete.

Prevention

A three-part strategy is the best way to prevent wound infections:

1. Identify patients at risk as outlined in Table 11-1.
2. Adhere to proper aseptic surgical techniques, including the use of skin antiseptic solutions, sterile instruments, handwashing, gloves, masks, and patient draping.
3. Use good surgical technique including gentle handling of tissue, minimize char and necrosis with electrocoagulation, tie sutures appropriately, and undermine at the proper tissue level.

At times, perioperative antibiotics may be employed to decrease the risk of infection. Some clinical circumstances that might warrant prophylactic antibiotics include elderly patients, insulin-dependent diabetes, significant kidney or liver disease, immunosuppression, and *S. aureus* carriers. In addition, a large, complex, or lengthy surgical procedure or a delayed closure of a wound may warrant antibiotics. Second-intention healing does not typically require treatment. Antibiotics for the purposes described above may be given prior to the surgical procedure and should be continued for a 1-week course. Erythromycin and penicillinase-resistant penicillins and cephalosporins are excellent choices for outpatient surgical procedures.

NECROSIS

Wound necrosis, or tissue death, results from circulatory compromise and tissue ischemia. An eschar of dead tissue forms, which eventually sloughs [Figure 11-8]. This slough may be superficial only (epidermal desquamation) or full thickness through the dermis. The most critical cause of tissue ischemia and necrosis is excessive tension on the wound edges. This can result from sutures being tied too tightly, insufficient or improper undermining, an expanding hematoma, infection-related edema and swelling, or wound edges that are simply pulled together under too much tension. Proper use of buried subcutaneous sutures will help reduce wound tension prior to placement of the epidermal sutures. Tissue with preexisting vascular compromise such as scar tissue or irradiated skin is also at increased risk for necrosis. Smokers are particularly at increased

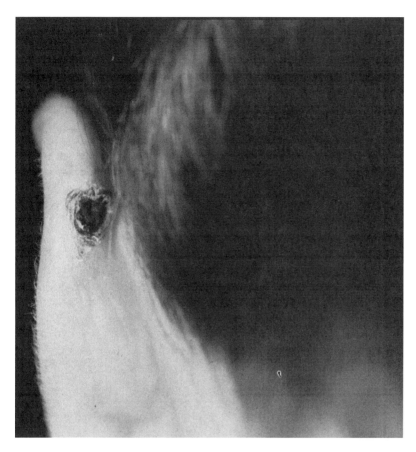

Figure 11-8. Necrosis
A small area of skin necrosis is noted in this flap performed on the upper helix. In general, areas of necrosis will slough and adequate skin will regrow in the area, resulting in a good cosmetic result. It is important to keep this area moist with antibiotic salve or petrolatum.

risk for tissue ischemia and necrosis, especially if skin grafts or flaps have been performed. Nicotine causes vasoconstriction, which may lower tissue oxygenation by more than 50%. In addition, carbon monoxide causes tissue hypoxia. The patient should be strongly encouraged to cease or reduce smoking 2–3 days prior to surgery and not commence smoking again for at least 5–7 days afterward.

➥ On the chest, shoulders, and back, avoid epidermal sutures. Well-placed buried sutures and Steri-Strips will be effective and will prevent the development of fang marks.

DEHISCENCE

Wound separation, or dehiscence, is usually due to infection or bleeding [Figure 11-9]. Both infection and bleeding can cause swell-

Surgical Complications

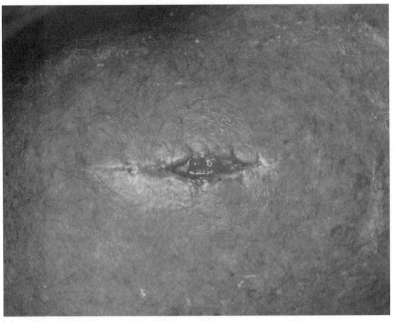

(a)

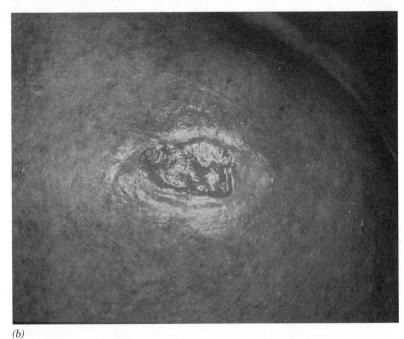

Figure 11-9. Wound Dehiscence
(a) A wound dehiscence as a result of tension or infection.
(b) The area is healing fully on its own. When wounds dehisce, it is important to assure the patient that the wound will heal in a satisfactory fashion. It is best if the wound is kept moist and covered.

(b)

ing, edema, and tension on the wound. Additionally, these complications may necessitate premature removal of sutures with resultant dehiscence. At times, direct trauma to the wound or excessive activity may result in wound dehiscence. Failure to use deep-layered sutures in areas of tension may result in dehiscence when the epidermal sutures are removed.

Bear in mind that at 1–2 weeks postoperatively, only 3–5% of the normal tensile strength of the wound has developed. Thus, the most vulnerable period for dehiscence is at suture removal, when tensile strength is still minimal. Skin closure tapes (Steri-Strips) will provide some support to the wound edges.

By 1 month, approximately 35% of the wound tensile strength will have redeveloped, allowing the wound to withstand the forces of most normal activity. This corresponds in time to the interval when buried subcutaneous sutures will be absorbed. By 6 months, 80% of the wound strength will have been achieved. Overzealous or premature jogging, swimming, weight lifting, aerobics, or contact sports may result in wound dehiscence.

The management of wound dehiscence depends on the causes and timing. A wound that opens cleanly due to trauma in the first 24 hours may be immediately resutured. Complicated dehiscence due to infection should heal by second-intention as should late dehiscence (after 24 hours) if resuturing is not desired.

OTHER POSTOPERATIVE PROBLEMS

Excess Granulation Tissue

Hypergranulation (proud flesh) typically occurs in wounds that heal by second intention. Hypergranulation tissue appears as spongy, pink-to-red tissue that covers the wound bed and extrudes above the surface [Figure 11-10]. It represents an overgrowth of fibroblasts and endothelial cells, but its cause is unknown. It is best to remove this excess granulation tissue as its persistence will serve as a mechanical barrier, preventing the new epidermis from migrating over the wound.

➥ Excess granulation tissue is a common problem when wounds are allowed to heal by second indention. It can be treated with silver nitrate, 70% TCA, or curettage.

Proud flesh can be treated with direct application of 70% trichloroacetic acid or with silver nitrate sticks. It is sometimes more effective to mechanically debride the tissue with a curette and control the subsequent bleeding with pressure and aluminum chloride. The hypergranulation tissue can regrow, so the patient should be seen

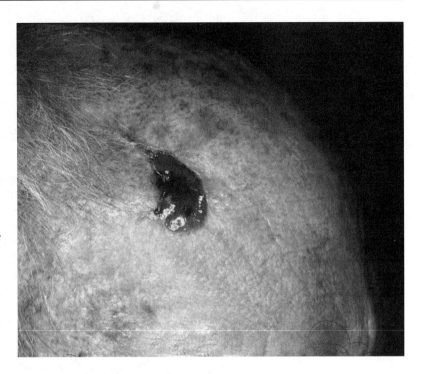

Figure 11-10. Granulation Tissue
So-called "proud flesh" or granulation tissue can develop especially when wounds are allowed to heal by second intention. Chemical cautery with 70% TCA or silver nitrate is effective and should be performed weekly until the area has resolved completely. Granulation tissue prevents the normal ingrowth of epidermis. Occasionally granulation tissue can be so dense that it must be curetted.

on a regular follow-up basis until reepithelialization of the wound is complete. Weekly visits are often sufficient.

Contact Dermatitis

A variety of agents used in the perioperative setting can cause allergic reactions [Figure 11-11]. Topical antibiotics are frequently used on the postoperative wound and can be a common cause of contact dermatitis. The most common sensitizing agent is neomycin, but any topical antibiotic can be a sensitizer. These agents are frequently used together ("triple antibiotic ointment"), are mixed with preservative agents, and are readily available over-the-counter. The risk of developing contact dermatitis is enhanced because topical antibiotics are usually used under occlusion for up to a week or longer. The true value of an antibiotic ointment in preventing wound infections is not proven, and thus substituting white petrolatum or other similar ointments (Aquaphor) may be better, especially in the patient sensitive to these agents.

Other Postoperative Problems

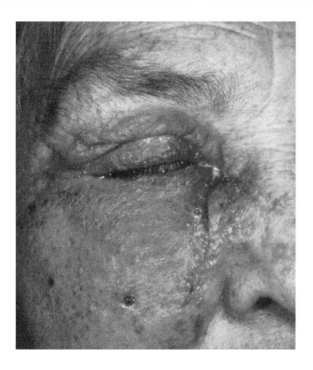

Figure 11-11. Allergic Reaction to Polysporin
Polysporin is a well-known sensitizer. This photograph demonstrates an allergic reaction to Polysporin that is as severe as a contact dermatitis from poison ivy. It may not be necessary to use antibiotic ointment at all as recent studies have demonstrated that Vaseline itself provides just as good protection against superficial wound infection.

Contact dermatitis manifests as a diffuse (corresponding to the area of application) erythematous patch, or plaque, which is often pruritic and frequently is studded with small, translucent vesicles. These findings can be mistaken for a wound infection, but the contact dermatitis is not tender or purulent. The presence of itching is very helpful in identifying a contact dermatitis. Treatment consists of discontinuing the offending agent and using a mid-strength topical steroid for several days.

Tape Reactions

Some patients may develop a simple irritant dermatitis to the adhesive in surgical tape, but others will have a severe allergic reaction with vesicle formation. Hypoallergenic paper tape can be helpful, but some patients will even react to this. In some locations, circumferential gauze or elastic wraps can hold the dressing in place, thus avoiding the use of adhesives.

➥ For patients who are allergic to Band-Aid adhesive, custom strips can be created with hypoallergenic tape and small squares of nonstick dressing.

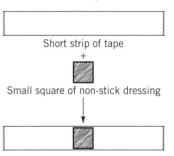

Skin Preparation Agents

Chlorhexidine gluconate (Hibiclens) is a popular surgical scrub because it causes minimal skin irritation and is a weak sensitizing agent. A few contact reactions to this agent have been reported. Povidone-iodine (Betadine) has a much higher incidence of contact allergies due to release of low concentrations of iodine. Phisoderm is an excellent surgical scrub with a low incidence of allergy. It has the added advantage of being safe for use around the eyes. Hibiclens has been reported to cause keratitis upon eye contact.

Latex Allergy

About 10% of persons are allergic to latex. Patients who are very sensitive to this compound can react to contact with the physician's gloved hand.

Scars

"What will my scar look like?" is the most common question people ask, but the most difficult to answer. Each person and each scar is highly individual and somewhat unpredictable. The final scar depends on so many factors, including anatomic location, age of the patient, skin elasticity, size and complexity of the surgical procedure, postoperative activity level, and skill of the surgeon. Patients must be warned about the formation of scars and potential adverse outcomes. It is well to point out that any surgery of the skin is, by definition, "plastic surgery," but this does not guarantee there will be "no scar."

➡ If a scar is persistently red, refer the patient for pulsed dye laser.

THICK SCARS. A hypertrophic scar is a thickened, raised scar that does not extend beyond the margins of the wound. It occurs most commonly in high tension areas such as the breasts, chest, upper back, and shoulders. Treatment consists of manual massage of the scar, injection with intralesional steroids, silicone sheeting and, some suggest, the pulsed dye laser. Manual massage can be extremely helpful to soften up scars. Light massage of the scar for 5–10 minutes two to three times a day will help remodel the collagen. The pressure must be onto a hard bony surface and the digital motion should be equivalent to kneading bread.

Intralesional triamcinolone is probably the most effective treatment for hypertrophic scars. It will help to flatten the scar and also alleviate any associated pruritus. Start injections at 3–5 mg/cc and increase to 10–20 mg/cc depending on the site of the scar and its thickness. Advise the patient of the risk of atrophy and telangiectasias.

Silicone sheeting is a relatively new treatment in which silicone-impregnated gel sheeting is applied directly to the wound. It is often used for weeks to months and seems to be most beneficial for new hypertrophic scars.

A keloid is an excessive scar that extends beyond the borders of the surgical site (see p. 219). Keloids can be very large and quite difficult to treat. They are, in fact, benign tumors of scar tissue. Excising the keloid may result in an even larger keloid. Intralesional steroids are probably the safest and most effective approach. It may be necessary to use 40 mg/cc triamcinolone. Pretreatment of the lesion with cryosurgery, followed by a 20-minute wait, will improve penetration of the steroid into the dense, unyielding mass of scar tissue. Pressure earrings at the site of treated earlobe keloids can also be helpful. More aggressive treatment of keloids including carbon dioxide laser ablation and radiation treatments may help but the recurrence rate is disappointingly high.

SPREAD SCARS. Scars can widen over time due to the forces of tension. Wide scars can develop where there is significant tension such as the shoulders, chest, and upper back, regardless of the degree of undermining at the time of closure. Scar spread may be minimized by using deep buried sutures and limiting heavy physical activity postoperatively.

PIGMENTARY CHANGE. Scars may develop hyper- or hypopigmentation. The ideal final result of most sutured wounds is a fine, white, linear line. The initial scar can be quite pink in color, sometimes for up to 4–6 months, and will slowly turn white. Patients with fair skin may stay pinker for a longer period of time. Some scars will initially hyperpigment, but most will assume a white color.

TELANGIECTASIAS. As scars mature, cosmetically noticeable telangiectatic vessels may appear, especially along the periphery of the surgical site. This seems most common in the central face, especially the nose and malar cheeks. The exact cause is unknown, but may be related to wound tension, skin type, and neovascularization. Treatment is best performed with the pulsed dye or copper vapor laser. For smaller telangiectatic vessels, a fine epilating needle with the Hyfrecator adjusted to a low setting can be quite effective.

Surgical Complications

EDEMA. Swelling of the surgical site is usually short term, but at times can be a chronic problem. Lower eyelid edema can take months to resolve. Long-term swelling of the digits and lower extremities can also occur.

SPITTING STITCH. A small percentage of patients will have a deep buried absorbable suture extrude from the surgical site. This can occur 3–6 weeks postoperatively, depending on the type of suture used. The cause of the spitting stitch is unclear. Patients are usually concerned about a late postoperative infection because the spitting stitch will often be associated with a small pustule. They can be reassured that treatment, which is the simple removal of the extrud-

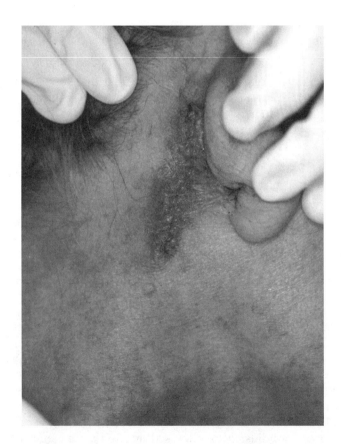

Figure 11-12. Suture Reaction
An allergic suture reaction to catgut is demonstrated here with erythema, inflammation, and swelling. It must be distinguished from a spitting suture, which is manifested either as a small pimple approximately 4 weeks after surgery or as a small bit of suture that can be seen poking through the skin like grass through pavement. In the latter case, the suture can easily be removed with prompt resolution of the problem. Alternatively, in the former case, the reaction will resolve only as the material itself resorbs.

ing material, will solve the problem. Encourage the patient to call you if he or she notices a spitting suture, because festering foreign matter may lead to an unsightly nubbin of scar tissue. A spitting suture is different than the irritant or allergic reaction that might develop early on from catgut sutures [Figure 11-12].

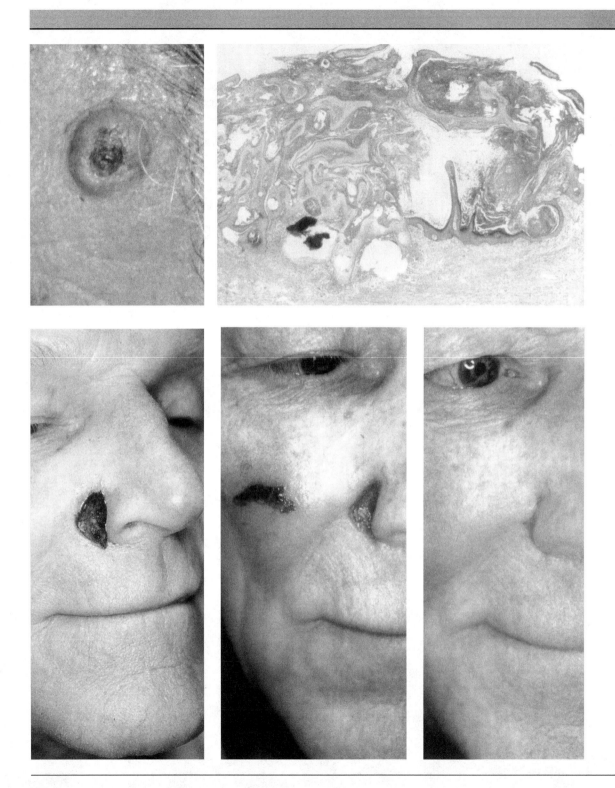

12

Special Topics in Dermatologic Surgery

In the realm of dermatologic surgery there are several special problems that are frequently encountered. A synopsis of practical approaches to these clinical challenges follows.

MELANOMA

Malignant melanoma is an increasingly common, lethal form of skin cancer. Any physician caring for patients should be able to make the clinical diagnosis of malignant melanoma. Although a lesion can be suspected on clinical grounds, the diagnosis can only be made definitively in the office by biopsy. Figure 12-1 demonstrates the range of appearance of malignant melanoma. Malignant melanoma must be diagnosed early because the cure rate for this lethal cancer is directly proportional to its depth of invasion at the time of diagnosis [Table 12-1]. Depth of invasion is usually related to the duration of the lesion. As a general rule, any pigmented lesion that has demonstrated a change in color, shape, size, which itches or bleeds (although those are late signs), or which the patient is concerned about, should be biopsied.

It is part of the subtlety of medicine that the patient often has an uncanny knowledge of what lesions are abnormal and should

➥ When doing an excisional biopsy in which the orientation of the specimen will be important to the pathologist, place the suture in the specimen, in situ, that is, before you have removed it completely.

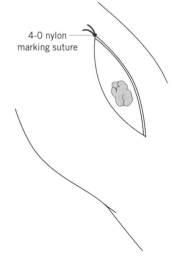

4-0 nylon marking suture

be addressed. It is not uncommon for a patient to highlight a lesion that appears to be of minimal concern to the dermatologist but upon biopsy indeed reveals either a melanoma, melanoma in situ or atypical nevus. For this reason, it is our policy that if a patient expresses concern about a lesion, through explicit verbal communication or some other hint, the lesion must be biopsied.

Many physicians state that they are unwilling to biopsy lesions on the face because they are worried about scars. In fact, when biopsying a lesion to rule out malignancy most patients believe the cosmetic result is secondary.

Physician experience with the lesion is paramount. This is especially the case with melanoma, where it is important to understand the histologic behavior of the lesion. It is not uncommon to see

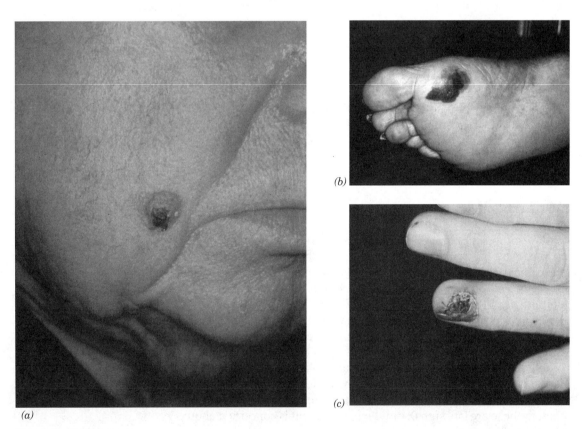

Figure 12-1. Melanoma
(a) Nodular melanoma. (b) Acral melanoma. This represents a serious lesion and is seen most commonly in non-Caucasian patients. (c) Advanced digital melanoma mistaken for a wart for many years.

TABLE 12-1 Five- and Ten-Year Survival Data for Prognostic Factors in 1130 Patients with Malignant Melanoma

Variables	Number of Patients	5-Year Survival (%)	10-Year Survival (%)
All patients	1130	87	79
Lesion thickness			
0–0.75 mm	320	99	98
0.76–1.69 mm	296	94	89
1.7–3.59 mm	253	81	67
3.6 mm or larger	147	49	43
No. of lymph nodes positive for tumor at regional lymph node dissection			
0	484	89	80
1	49	53	32
2–3	32	39	21
4 or more	25	31	10
Histologic type			
Lentigo maligna melanoma	43	92	85
Superficial spreading MM	802	91	83
Nodular MM	101	62	57
Acral lentiginous MM	35	79	68
Anatomic site			
Head and neck	168	82	73
Trunk	411	84	75
Upper extremity	195	94	87
Lower extremity	245	93	86
Acral	88	83	73
High risk	182	77	67
Intermediate risk	750	87	80
Low risk	166	96	90
Age			
Less than 50	506	90	84
50 or older	624	84	75
Gender			
Female	578	90	84
Male	550	83	74
Ulceration			
Absent	792	91	84
Present	188	71	59
Regression			
Present	184	95	87
Absent	638	85	77

Source: Adapted from Friedman, R. J. et al., 1991, *Cancer of the Skin*, Saunders, Philadelphia.

TABLE 12-2 Margins of Excision

Diagnosis	Margin (cm)
Atypical nevus	.3–.5
Lentigo maligna	.5
Melanoma up to 1 mm in depth	1
1.0–2.0 mm	2
>2.0 mm	3

seborrheic keratoses, which are benign superficial epidermal lesions, removed with full-thickness excision. This results in a permanent linear scar when in fact a gentle curettage would have resulted in a superb cosmetic outcome with complete elimination of the lesion. It is axiomatic in dermatology that microscopically superficial lesions be treated with superficial methods.

Management

The management of melanoma is an example of the sad truth that old habits die hard. The original treatment of melanoma evolved in the early 1900s as the result of a single case report by Handley, an English surgeon. He performed an autopsy on a single patient with melanoma and determined that melanoma cells were present within 5 cm of the original lesion. It was on this basis that the original view developed that melanoma could be cured only with 5 cm margins. This attitude, which resulted in aggressive surgery regardless of location and which, when one reviews the literature, actually has no substantiation in fact, persists even to this day among physicians not particularly knowledgeable about melanoma. With the passage of time we have been able to learn from several prospective studies.

➡ When biopsying a suspicious lesion for melanoma, be certain to sample the full depth of the lesion.

The aggressiveness of melanoma and its risk of metastasis is related first and foremost to its depth measured in millimeters at the time of diagnosis. This is the Breslow depth. Historically, Clark's level, a measurement of the depth of invasion based on the microscopic substructure of the skin, has been cited but is not thought to be as predictive as Breslow depth.

Melanoma up to 1 mm in depth has a 98% 5 year cure rate with simple office excision of the primary lesion. Melanoma 1–2 mm in depth have a very high 5-year survival rate as well. Melanomas greater than 3 mm have a high risk of metastasis. The deeper the melanoma, the greater access it has to the lymphatics of the dermis and subcutis.

Excision of these lesions correlates with the anticipated degree of aggressiveness and the risk of in-transit metastases. Melanomas up to 1 mm can be excised with 1 cm margins, no more, no less. In situ melanoma can be excised with 0.5 cm margins. A melanoma 1–2 mm in depth can be adequately excised with 2 cm margins (Table 12-2). The data with respect to larger excision margins on lesions deeper than 3 mm are not yet conclusive. The issue of the role of lymphadenectomy for melanoma—which previously had been done on a routine basis—is undergoing reappraisal and it is best to discuss the issue with the oncologic surgeon.

In the case of a high-risk melanoma, the patient should be referred to a medical oncologist with expertise in melanoma.

LENTIGO MALIGNA

A condition associated with malignant melanoma is lentigo maligna. It is seen primarily in older individuals and consists of a variegated hyperpigmented patch on the cheek that can be present for many years [see Figure 12-3]. This lesion consists of malignant melanocytes confined to the epidermis and is analogous to squamous cell carcinoma in situ. In this sense it is a noninvasive lesion. However, the concern about lentigo maligna is that it can eventually, over many years, evolve into invasive melanoma [Figure 12-2]. Moreover, when this happens, especially if the lentigo maligna has been treated, the invasive melanoma can be difficult to diagnose and may even take the form of desmoplastic melanoma or melanoma in scar.

Lentigo maligna can be treated by staged excision if it is too large for a single procedure. Skin grafting and repair by flap can be problematic because of the high likelihood of marginal recurrence. It is therefore important to have all skin specimens reviewed by a skilled dermatopathologist. In this day of managed care, it is likely that you will have to jump through many hurdles to have your specimens read by a competent dermatopathologist, but the patient's life can often depend on it.

Cryosurgery is another approach to the management of lentigo maligna. In this case, there is a risk of recurrent disease under the scar tissue, which may represent invasive melanoma and may not be diagnosed until the lesion has become advanced.

➤ When excising a pigmented lesion, always study it first with a Wood's light and mark the margins prior to anesthetizing.

Special Topics in Dermatologic Surgery

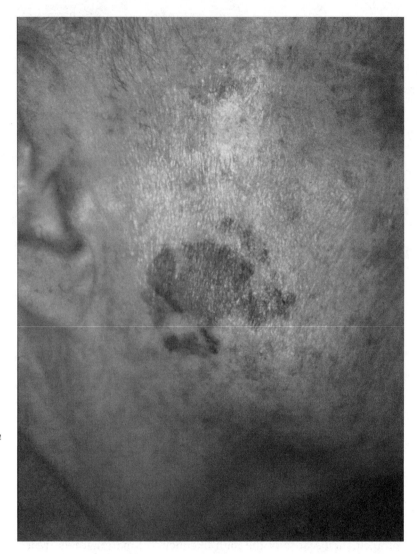

Figure 12-2. Lentigo Maligna Melanoma
An invasive melanoma developed in the presence of longstanding lentigo maligna. These lesions are challenging to treat because of their large surface area.

NEVI

The diagnosis and management of nevi can be especially complex. Many lesions appear to be nevi that are really not, and only a skilled physician can tell the difference. Many nevi that appear atypical and may be precursors for melanoma are, in fact, not. Similarly,

TABLE 12-3 Clinical Characteristics of Nevocytic Nevi (NN)/Malignant Melanoma (MM)

Feature	Nondysplastic Nevocytic Nevus	Dysplastic Nevocytic Nevus	Malignant MM
Size	Usually <6 mm	Often >7 mm	Often >6 mm
Uniformity (when multiple)	Homogeneous	Heterogeneous	Heterogeneous
Number	Few (10–40) NN	Often many NN (>50–100)	Usually 1 MM
Perimeter	Regular	Irregular (±); indistinct	Irregular
Color	Uniform	Usually variegated	Usually variegated
Hue	Tan, brown	Tan-brown-black-red	Tan-brown-black-red-white-blue
"Shoulder"	Uncommon	Almost always	Often
Symmetry	Symmetric	Symmetric (±)	Asymmetric
Elevation	Macular to nodular	Usually papular to plaque centrally	Macular plaque to nodular
Hypertrichosis	Uncommon	None	None
Erosion/ulceration	None	None	May be present
Location	Usually trunk > limbs	Usually trunk > limbs > head	Men: trunk > limbs; Women: limbs > trunk
Symptoms	Usually none	Usually none	Often
Change	Slow then stable	Slow then stable	Faster/continuous
Surrounding skin	Normal	Normal	May have satellites/sun damage

Source: Adapted from Friedman, R. J. et al., 1991, *Cancer of the Skin*, Saunders, Philadelphia.

often benign-appearing lesions can evolve into melanoma, which is especially worrisome even for the most skilled dermatologist. Some guidelines are presented in Table 12-3. If a diagnosis of a benign nevus has been made, it can be excised either by the tangential technique or full thickness and closed with sutures. Atypical nevi should be photographically documented and the biopsy should always be read by a skilled dermatopathologist. When indicated, congenital nevi may be excised in a staged fashion if they are too large for primary closure [Figure 12-3]. Patients with multiple atypical nevi and their affected relatives should be followed by a dermatologist with special interest in pigmented lesions.

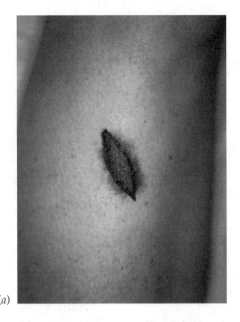

(a)

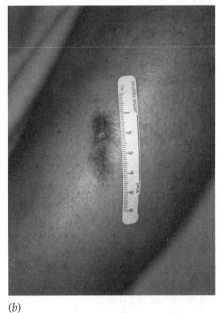

(b)

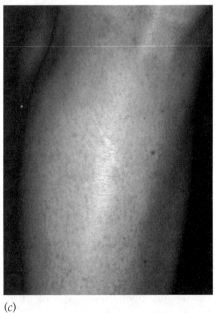

(c)

Figure 12-3. Staged Excision
(a) Nevus on anterior shin is present in a location which is normally difficult to excise and close primarily. To minimize the scar, staged excision is preferable to excision with skin grafting. Design and mark your ellipse including the maximal amount of tissue that can be excised and closed primarily. (b) Healed site after first stage excision of nevus at approximately three months postop. Re-excision of the residual nevus can now be performed using an elliptical excision with side-to-side closure. (c) Follow up at nine months after complete excision of congenital nevus. Note minimal scar.

SKIN CANCER

Basal Cell Cancer

Basal cell cancer is the most common form of human cancer. Increasingly, it is occurring in younger patients. This is likely caused by changes in lifestyle and increased exposure to ultraviolet radiation during leisure time. There are several different clinical subtypes of basal cell cancer and all should be recognized. A common mistake is to diagnose a superficial basal cell cancer as a patch of eczema. Tragic outcomes have occurred where a misdiagnosis led to treatment with topical steroids. As a general rule, if a lesion does not improve with topical steroids after 2 weeks, it should be biopsied.

Basal cell cancer can be treated in a variety of ways. The simplest method is electrodesiccation and curettage. In this procedure the area is infiltrated with lidocaine and epinephrine and a disposable curette is used to debulk the tissue and the edge around the tumor. Light cautery is then applied. Although the traditional approach consists of electrocautery and curettage for three cycles, superficial basal cell cancer is easily treated with just one cycle of curettage properly performed without necessarily cauterizing the site. This will minimize scar formation. Deep nodular basal cell cancers and other clinical subtypes should be excised.

Squamous Cell Cancer

Squamous cell cancer (SCC) of the skin is also increasing in incidence. It presents on the head and neck, and although more often seen in men, it is being diagnosed in women as well. SCC does have the potential to metastasize, especially when it is greater than 1 cm and occurs on the ear, temple, or lip. It should be treated by excision, Mohs' surgery, or radiation where indicated by extent of tumor or the patient's medical condition.

A specific subtype of squamous cell cancer is keratoacanthoma [Figure 12-4]. This is a crater-form nodular lesion that develops in a rapid period (approximately over 2 months) and historically has been said to regress on its own. Dermatologists have often taken a conservative approach, including radiation or injectable antineoplastic agents. When keratoacanthoma occurs in the central face, it is at risk for behaving in a very aggressive fashion, even leading to metastasis and death. Central facial keratoacanthoma should be considered a squamous cell cancer and treated in an aggressive fashion.

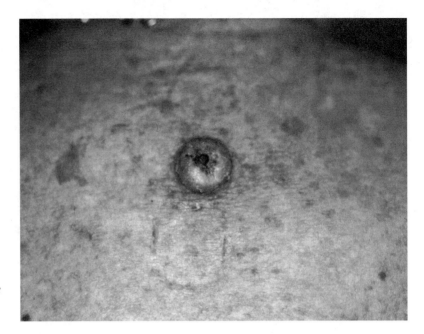

Figure 12-4. Keratoacanthoma
This rapidly growing lesion is often considered to be benign, but in fact represents a variant of squamous cell carcinoma. In the central facial area it has the potential for extreme destruction or even metastasis.

MOHS' SURGERY

Mohs' microscopically controlled excision is a specialized form of surgery for the treatment of basal cell cancer and squamous cell cancer. It is also occasionally used for some rare skin malignancies. Although small primary lesions are easily excised with the techniques described in this book, the meticulous Mohs' method provides the highest cure rate for histologically and clinically aggressive lesions and lesions with other challenging characteristics [Figure 12-5].

The Mohs' technique is usually indicated for recurrent nonmelanoma skin cancer, primary basal cell cancer in individuals where cosmesis is a major concern, and cancer near free margins such as the eyelids or lips. The embryonic fusion plane or central facial areas are also of special concern because incompletely treated cancers in these areas have a high risk of recurrence with deep extension. The Mohs' technique is cost efficient if performed by a physician who specializes in the technique on a routine basis.

Mohs' surgery was originally developed by Frederick Mohs in the 1940s when he was a medical student at the University of Wisconsin. His original description of the procedure involved the applica-

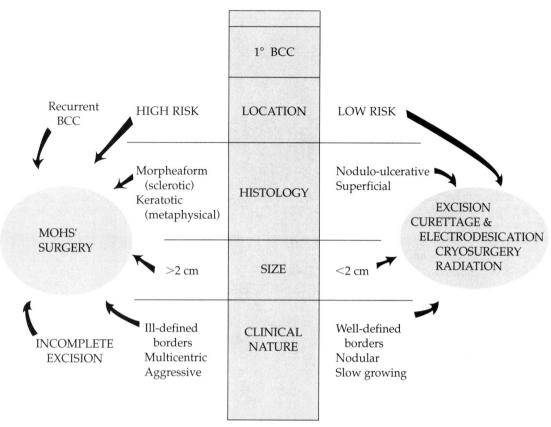

Figure 12-5. Mohs' Algorithm
The approach to performing Mohs' surgery is outlined here. There are many different approaches to the management of skin cancer. It is important to identify those that are high risk and require Mohs' surgery. Chart courtesy of Neil A. Swanson, M.D.

tion of zinc chloride paste to tissue. The tissue fixed in situ, and after it was removed the next day as a thin layer, the specimen was carefully mapped out so that one could return to the patient and remove any residual cancer without being additionally aggressive. This technique, which tended to be painful and resulted in defects that healed by second intention, was termed *chemosurgery*. Unfortunately, that term is still used today by physicians not fully familiar with the modern version of the technique.

The Mohs' surgery technique, also referred to as microscopically controlled excision, is currently performed in a rapid fashion using horizontal frozen sections [Figure 12-6]. It is not *chemo*surgery. The advantage of the Mohs' technique is that it is cost-efficient, tissue sparing, and highly curative. Because cure of nonmelanoma skin

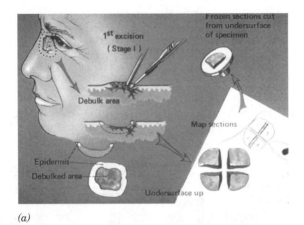

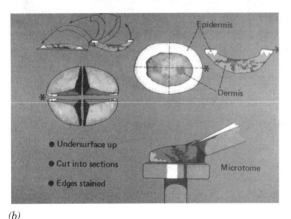 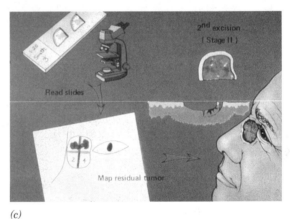

Figure 12-6. Mohs' Surgery
Mohs' surgery demonstrated in its sequential fashion. Illustrations courtesy of Neil A. Swanson, M.D.

cancer does not require an extra margin of tissue, as does melanoma, extirpation of the tumor alone is sufficient if all histologic margins have been cleared. Traditional methods of assessing surgical margins are adequate with nodular basal cell carcinoma and other limited lesions. Various subtypes of basal cell cancer, however, such as aggressive-growth basal cell cancer, have digitate growth and complete margin analysis is not possible by conventional methods. The Mohs' technique allows excision of the tumor in a tissue-sparing fashion and evaluation of all the margins 360 degrees around.

The definition of Mohs' surgery is quite specific. It requires that the physician excising the tumor be the one who maps it and interprets the tissue specimen as well. The Mohs' surgeon is simultaneously acting as surgeon and pathologist. It is this combined effort that likely reduces the chance for error in map identification and tumor localization.

Following Mohs' surgery, the patient is tumor-free, and the wound can be immediately reconstructed or allowed to heal by second intention. Wounds may be allowed to heal by second intention when they are in concave areas. Although most Mohs' surgeons are trained in plastic reconstruction techniques, they also work in close association with plastic surgeons and facial plastic surgeons who may then take over the reconstructive aspects of especially complicated cases.

CYSTS

Epidermal cysts are a common presenting complaint. They are easily removed in office surgery. When a patient presents with an inflamed cyst that appears to have ruptured or become infected, it is best not to operate immediately. Ten mg per cc intralesional Kenalog should be injected and the patient should be advised to use warm compresses. Antibiotics may be prescribed. Dramatic reduction in the size of the cyst may then occur. Once the cyst has been quiescent for a reasonable amount of time, one should excise the residual lesion, which is at high risk for recurrence. This is best done by infiltrating the area with lidocaine and epinephrine and making a small incision through the pore (which is the opening of the cyst). While applying pressure on either side of the cyst so that the skin overlying it is taut, gently score the incision slowly until the cyst's sac can be seen [Figure 12-7]. Once this is noted, use a skin hook to gently dissect around the cyst itself.

It is not uncommon for the cyst to rupture and eject a substantial amount of foul-smelling cheesy material. If this should happen, one must be certain to have the wound clear of this debris as it can stimulate an inflammatory reaction. However, if the cyst is kept intact, the procedure can be completed by gently dissecting and, while applying gentle pressure around the cyst, observing it to pop out.

Excision of pilar cysts, which are a form of epidermoid inclusion cysts of the scalp, is much easier because these more thickly walled

Special Topics in Dermatologic Surgery

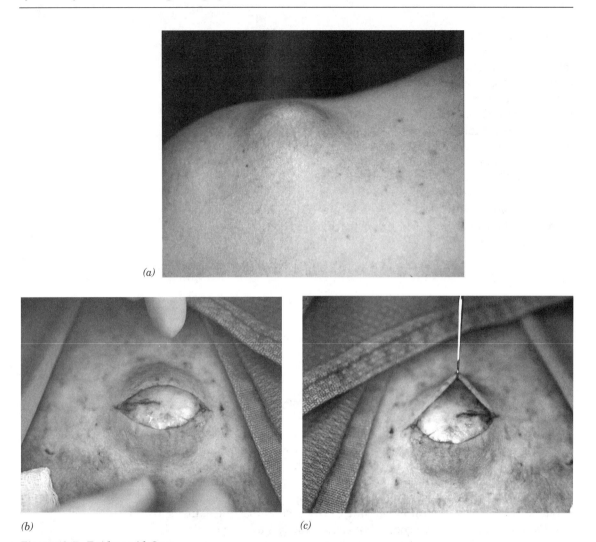

Figure 12-7. Epidermoid Cyst
(a) Epidermoid cyst. (b) Infiltration of the cyst area with copious amounts of lidocaine and gentle incision over the cyst. Careful dissection around the cyst often permits removal without expression of contents. In cases where one would like to minimize the incision and the cyst has not been previously ruptured, so no scar tissue is present, it is reasonable to make a small incision after the cyst has been mobilized, express the contents, and then remove the sac itself.

lesions tend to rupture less frequently and can often be removed en bloc. The wound can then be closed with a buried suture or simple interrupted 6-0 Prolene sutures if the skin is thin and the cyst has been relatively superficial.

KELOIDS AND SCARS

Despite the best efforts of the physician, certain patients will demonstrate a tendency to develop hypertrophic scars and keloids [Figure 12-8]. In addition, patients may also develop spread scars in areas of great tension, or subsequent to dehiscence from trauma or poor technique.

Keloids are among the most difficult lesions to manage. A first-line approach is to use cryosurgery and intralesional steroids. The keloid should be treated with one or two aggressive freeze/thaw cycles of liquid nitrogen so that the keloid becomes swollen. The swelling stretches the scar fibers and permits better penetration of the steroid. Ten to forty mg per cc Kenalog should be used, despite the attendant risk of thinning of the skin. This should be repeated every 4 weeks for at least 6 months and the patient should be closely observed. There has been much discussion of the use of silicone gel sheeting (SGS). This particular topical dressing, which is reusable, is of benefit in the case of some early scars but will have no benefit in the case of a mature keloid. In general, SGS tends to have a smoothing effect on the scar and is active only when the dressing is used. Many patients find this inconvenient and the benefits not sufficient to warrant the nuisance of regular use.

LIPOMAS

Lipomas can be easily removed with a 4–6 mm skin punch. These encapsulated lesions are often quite large but compressible. For this reason, it is not justifiable to make a large incision for the removal of a lesion that can be compressed through a relatively small hole. After making your punch incision, remove the core and gently compress the limpoma while working around the capsule through the hole with a small hemostat. Eventually the lipoma will pop out and the wound can be closed with one or two sutures.

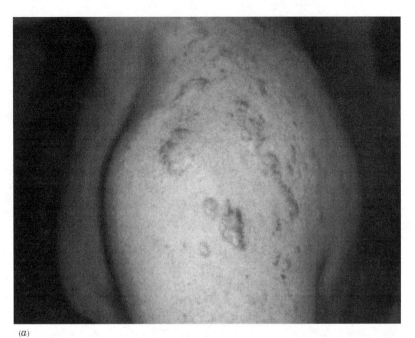

(a)

Figure 12-8. Keloid and Hypertrophic Scars
(a) Keloids can develop in response to any trauma, whether surgical or other. Here, a patient with severe cystic acne is left with persistent keloids of the trunk. (b) A hypertrophic scar developing in a patient in whom a nevus has been removed. Note the streaking pigmentation within the scar tissue. This represents the nevus cell growing within the bands of scar tissue.

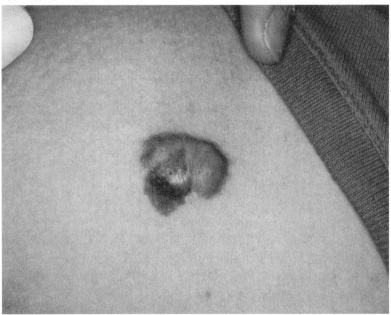

(b)

WHEN TO REFER

Although the procedures described in this book have been performed for generations by a whole range of physicians, there is no question that the complexity of dermatology may strain even the most highly skilled physician without special training in dermatology. Each physician, of course, must be guided by his or her own skill and comfort levels, but in general the following conditions should be referred to a dermatologist for thorough evaluation and management:

- Patients with atypical nevi
- Patients with family history of melanoma
- Patients with multiple basal cell skin cancers
- Patients with squamous cell carcinoma
- Patients with severe solar damage

The Action Guide in the Appendix may be helpful.

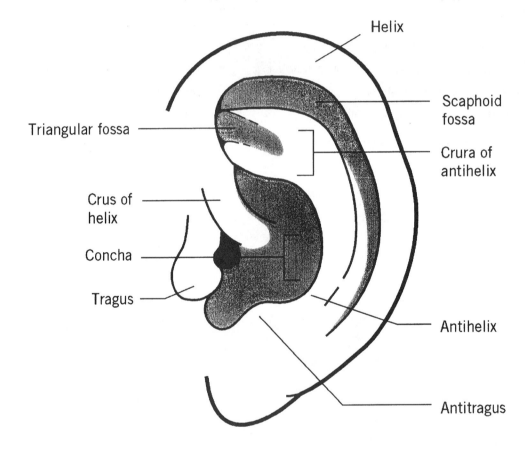

13

Risk Management

A regional discount clothing chain crows in advertisements that an educated consumer is their best customer. In medicine an informed individual will make your best patient. Patients who feel they have been educated about what is to happen to them heal faster and are generally more satisfied than patients who are less prepared. The need to obtain informed consent from patients should not be viewed as a burden but as an opportunity to enhance your communication and relationship with your patient. Should untoward events occur later, the foundation you will have built will serve you well.

Despite the advantage of the informed consent process, it is a regrettable fact of the modern practice of medicine that medical-legal considerations command an increasing amount of attention. Failure to diagnose is a very common cause of legal action and, in the world of dermatologic surgery, it is an important concern. But other issues arise as well. The procedures you perform during skin surgery will leave permanent scars apparent to all. This is distinct from invasive procedures such as sigmoidoscopy which, though they have their own risk, will not result in external, permanent changes. In the same vein, medical-legal risks associated with cosmetic procedures are different from those associated with surgical procedures of the skin performed to diagnose cancer. Rarely is a lawsuit initiated or won because of an unsatisfactory result secondary to a biopsy to diagnose cancer. However, an unsatisfactory result following a cosmetic skin procedure may initiate legal action.

This chapter describes the routine steps that should be taken in preparing the patient for surgery. You must always remember that the goal of any of the procedures described in this manual is the comprehensive care of the patient. Although it is best not to have to practice medicine defensively, there are several steps to take and specific attitudes you can develop that will allow you to do what is best for your patient and minimize any preoccupation with respect to risk management.

INFORMED CONSENT

There is much debate about the nature of informed consent. It is generally agreed that at a minimum, the diagnosis, treatment, alternative therapies, and related risks and benefits should be reviewed with the patient. In this context it is necessary to explain the impact of failure to treat. There are no clear guidelines about what you must tell your patients, although it is generally agreed that you are not required to review facts and issues that are common knowledge. For example, although it might be common knowledge that infection is a risk of surgery, gangrene with loss of a digit in a diabetic patient may not be. Historically, the physician's disclosure has been measured either by the *professional standard* or the *patient-oriented standard*. The former assumes that in sophisticated technical matters the physician is in the position to know what is best for the patient and can make judgments about how much information to share. In the latter standard, the physician must reveal all information that the patient would *need* to make a proper decision.

Ultimately, law and statutes are only imperfect guides. There is no substitute for good communication. You as a physician care about your patient, care about how the patient is managed, care about making a prompt diagnosis and want to cure in an effective and timely fashion. If the patient understands that these are your motives, the chance of lawsuit is usually low regardless of outcome. It is necessary, however, to fully inform the patient of the various risks and benefits associated with any of the procedures that you intend to pursue.

The issue of whether a patient understands what has been discussed is related to informed consent. Numerous studies have documented a recall rate of 10–30% when patients are asked, after giving informed consent, whether they remember the risks. Clearly there are many instances where patients have signed detailed informed consents and have later said in the context of a lawsuit that, yes, they signed it, but they did not really know what they were reading. In some cases, fear and anxiety may truly have prevented the patient from remembering what was being discussed. It is because of the mysteries of the human mind that a solid doctor–patient relationship is paramount. Sheaves of documents cannot patch up a relationship that was never properly cultivated.

After a patient presents in the office with a lesion that requires diagnosis, it is wise to explain why the lesion is of concern and what diagnosis would entail. Using a mirror, demonstrate to the patient the extent of the lesion, and ask if the patient concurs with the area of concern. It is important to do this because patients frequently present with a question about a lesion that is clinically of less concern than that upon which you focus. Occasionally the patient may say that he or she is not sure of the lesion, but after discussing it and reviewing the adjacent anatomic landmarks, you will invariably come to agreement about the site. After the lesion has been identified, explain to the patient that you will inject a local anesthetic and that it will sting. The "growth" or "spot" will either be shave excised or removed "through the full thickness of the skin and stitched." In either case, describe the type of scar that can be expected and emphasize that it is impossible to operate on the skin without getting some sort of scar. The important issue, you should hasten to add, is whether the scar will be noticeable. Take a few moments to discuss this and other complications with the patient. It is wise to emphasize that no surgeon in the world can do surgery on the skin without creating a scar. You might caution the patient that if he ever encounters a physician who says he can excise a lesion and leave no scar, he should get out of his office as quickly as possible.

One of the problems that we have when communicating with patients about scars is that the patient's conception of scar is different from ours. Our understanding is a biological one. We recognize that when tissue is injured it must repair itself and that the net result of that repair is something that is either minimally noticeable or, in an unfortunate situation at the other end of the spectrum, highly noticeable. Patients, however, conceive of the term *scar* in the context of *Phantom of the Opera*. For patients, scar has only negative connotations and, although you will never be able to change this conception on the part of the patient in the context of an office visit, it is important to emphasize that a scar is the result of a normal healing process and that individual tendencies will have as much impact on the final result as the skill of the surgeon. You might choose to highlight that a short scar can be very ugly or a lengthy scar can be so skillfully done that it is minimally noticeable. Although it is not always necessary to have this detailed a discussion about scarring, countless nights of sleep have been lost, never to be regained, by physicians who have operated on patients who believed they would have no scar. Ultimately, a few extra minutes spent discussing these issues with the patient will save many hours of aggravation later on. It is also reasonable to mention when obtaining informed consent that if there should be an unsatisfactory result from the biopsy or other procedure, certain refinements can be done in the future. After all aspects of the procedure have been discussed and the patient has been asked if she has any more questions, she is asked to sign a standard informed consent form [see Chapter 9, Figure 9-3].

DOCUMENTATION

Increasingly, documentation is the physician's second best defense against the trauma of legal assault. The first defense, of course, is good patient communication. It is important to document the essence of all the conversations that take place with the patient and document the procedure itself. (See Figure 13.1). Forms with check-off boxes are also extremely helpful to document discussions, and if prepared with a noncarbon copy, the patient may take a copy home for review. These time-saving techniques meet all medical-legal requirements for documenting in detail the procedures that you have done and the consent you have obtained.

The range of documentation, even among specialists in skin disease, is certainly remarkable. It is not unheard of to see records of melanoma treatment where a simple sentence and sketchy diagnosis have been entered into the chart. It is better to be detailed with documentation and assure everyone in posterity will be able to understand exactly what you did than to skimp and leave room for question about your technique, thoroughness, or competence. By the same token, excessive detail documenting informed consent may not be appropriate as it implies that you made an effort to convey every possible outcome when this, of course, *is* a practical impossibility.

It is important to have a system for tracking biopsies and arranging for follow-up. If a patient fails to return for treatment of a medically necessary problem, document this in his chart and send him a letter, return receipt guaranteed, explaining that (a) he did not show up for an appointment, (b) his condition needs treatment, and (c) if he does not want you to treat him, you will be happy to forward his records to a physician of his choice.

Operative Report

Date: _____
Patient Name: _____
Patient DOB: _____
Surgeon   Ellen Jones, M.D.
Assistant: _____
Nurse: _____

Anesthesia: Local with lidocaine   Lidocaine 1% with epi   Other_____

Preoperative Diagnosis: _____

Preoperative procedure: Excision with layered plastic closure

Indications: The patient is a _____ year old <u>man</u>   <u>woman</u> who presents with a _____ of the _____ which has been present for _____. Complete excision is indicated because _____. The risks and benefits of surgery were discussed with the patient and opportunity to ask questions was provided. After informed consent was obtained the patient was prepared for surgery.

Procedure: The patient was placed <u>supine</u>   <u>prone</u> on the operating suite table. The lesion was identified, the excision outlined mark and anesthetized with ____ cc of anesthetic solution as noted above. After complete anesthesia was obtained and the patient was prepped and draped, a full thickness excision along the previously marked lines was performed. Hemostasis was obtained with electrocautery. The specimen was sent to pathology after the margins were marked with suture. The wound edges were then undermined bluntly as needed and hemostasis was again obtained. The wound edges were approximated with _____ buried suture. The epidermis was then approximated with _____ <u>simple</u>   <u>interrupted</u>   <u>running</u> sutures. The final wound length was ____ cms. The wound was cleansed and dressed with a sterile pressure dressing. The patient will return in _____ days for _____.

Final diagnosis: _____
Final procedure: Excision with layered plastic closure
Complications: None
Operative Time: _____

_____
Ellen Jones, M.D.

Figure 13.1 Sample Operative Report
Documentation of surgery is critical. For convenience you may develop a series of operative reports that you can complete at time of surgery by filling in the blanks or circling options (e.g., underlined words above). If forms are prepared as noncarbon sets, one copy can be sent to the insurance company and the original retained in the chart.

CONFIDENTIALITY

The protection of confidentiality is what distinguishes physicians from many other professionals. The expectation of confidentiality is the first clause in the unwritten contract between patient and doctor. Patient confidentiality must be respected at all times. This includes the office setting itself where discussion of patients can be overheard and it applies to what information is provided to physicians who are not directly involved with the patient's care.

Good intentions provide no legal protection. Patient confidentiality must be an absolute. This will increasingly distinguish physicians from the unlicensed medical practitioners—insurance company employees—who now control vast masses of "confidential" patient information but are bound by no legal or moral constraints to protect it.

In summary, the best offense is a good defense. Keep the lawyer out of your office and the patients in it by remembering that good rapport with your patients is essential. Most problems in communication result from (1) not responding to patient questions, (2) not being available, and (3) appearing not to care. Avoid these pitfalls and you will likely sleep better at night knowing your patients are informed and educated.

APPENDIX I

Action Guides

SKIN BIOPSY
PIGMENTED LESIONS
BASAL CELL CANCER
SQUAMOUS CELL CANCER
COMPLICATIONS

These action guides are intended to give a general outline on how to approach common dermatologic problems. The pathways provided in these guides are not intended to accommodate variations in specific cases and circumstances where individual judgment should be the final arbiter.

Appendix I

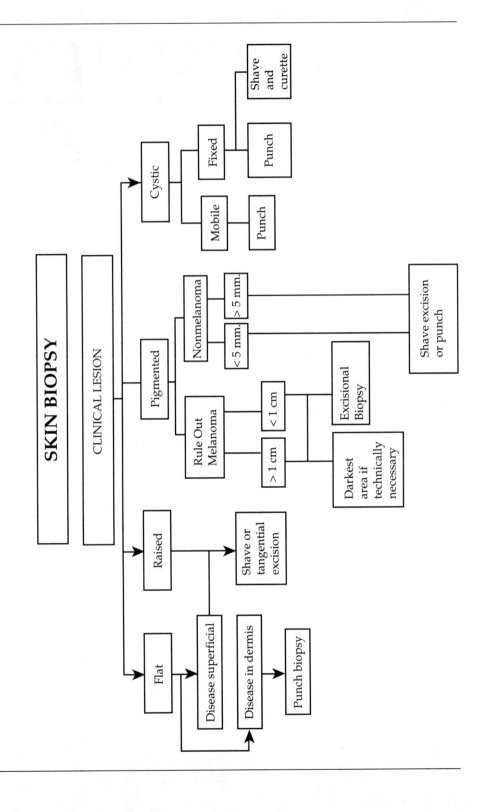

Appendix I

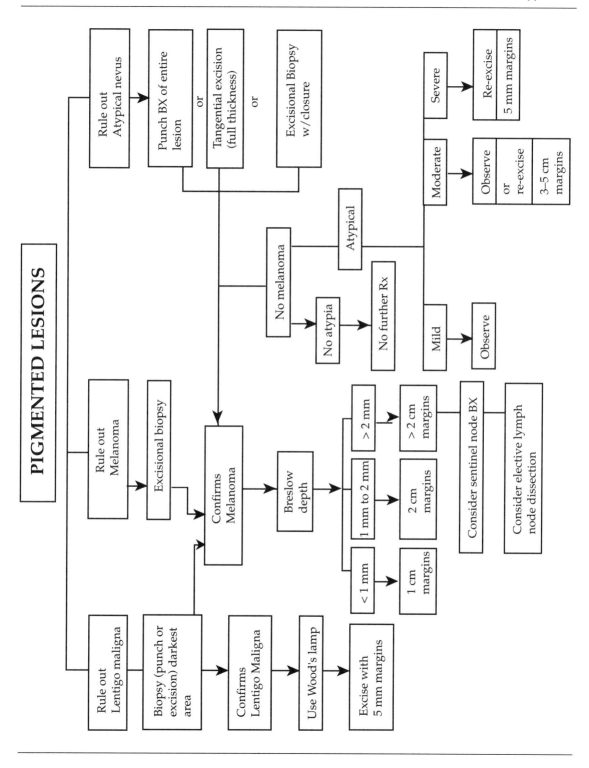

231

Appendix I

BASAL CELL CANCER

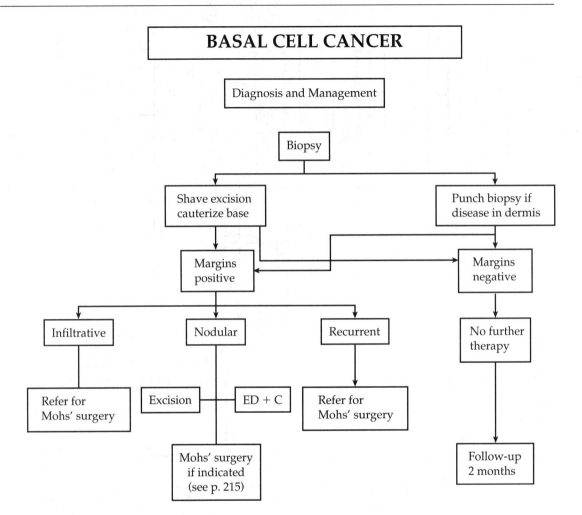

Appendix I

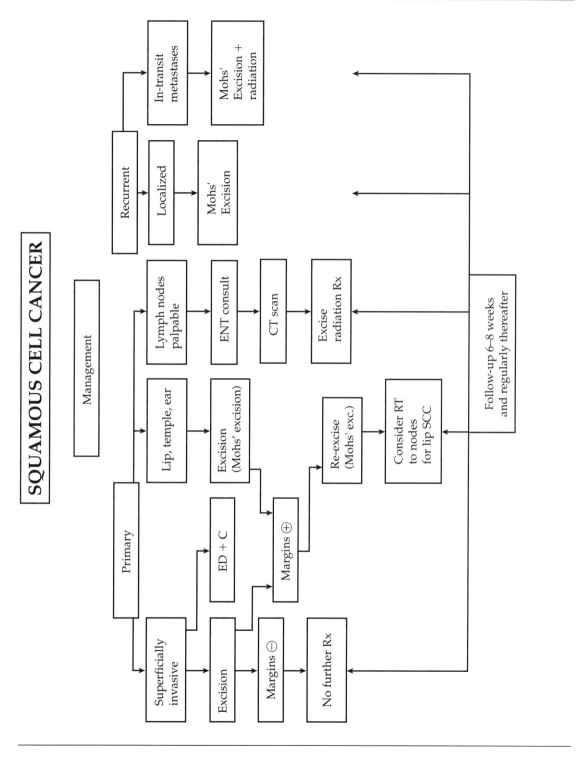

233

Appendix I

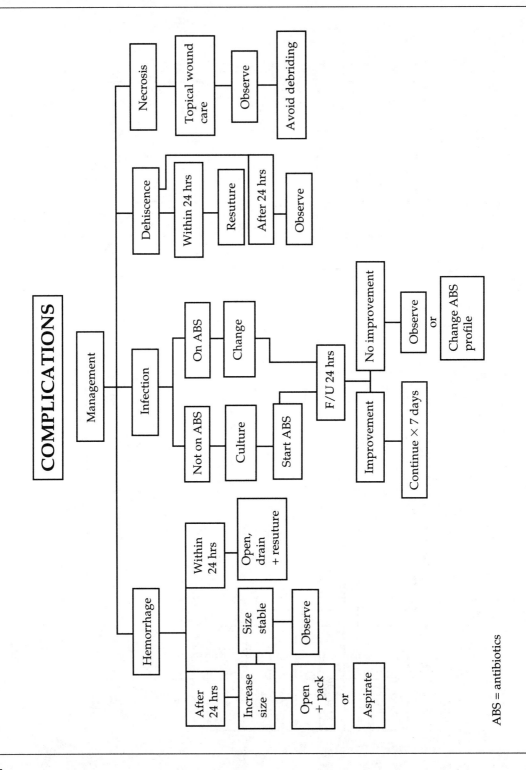

APPENDIX II

Vendors for Dermatologic Surgery Suite

INSTRUMENTS

Arista Surgical Supply Company
67 Lexington Avenue
New York, NY 10010

Bernsco Surgical Supply Company
6653 N.E. Windermere Road
Seattle, WA 98115

Miltex Instruments Company, Inc.
Ohio Drive
Lake Success, NY 11042

Robbins Instruments, Inc.
2 North Passaic Avenue
Catham, NJ 07928

George Tiemann & Company
84 Newtown Plaza
Plainview, NY 11803

OPERATING ROOM CHAIR

DMI
Division of Health Chair
  Corporation
2601 S. Constitution Boulevard
Salt Lake City, UT 84119

Midmark Corporation
60 Vista Drive
Versailles, OH 45380

CAUTERY

Birtcher Corporation
4501 North Arden Drive
El Monte, CA 91731

**Ellman International
  Manufacturing, Inc.**
Ellman Building
1136 Railroad Avenue
Hewlett, NY 11557

ULTRASONIC CLEANERS

ESMA Chemicals, Inc.
P.O. Box 162
Highland Park, IL 60035

SUTURES

Davis and Geck
Division of American Cyanamid
  Co.
One Cyanamid Plaza
Wayne, NJ 07470

Ethicon, Inc.
Route 22
Somerville, NJ 08876

ADHESIVE AGENT

Mastisol
Ferndale Labs, Inc.
780 W. Eight Mile Road
Ferndale, MI 48220

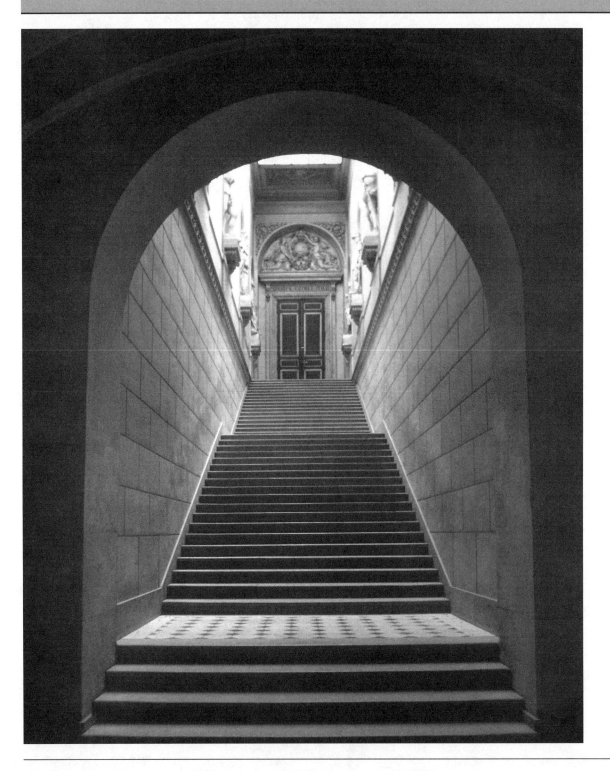

Further Reading

Skin Surgery. Ervin Epstein and Ervin Epstein, Jr., W. B. Saunders Co., Philadelphia, PA, 1987.
This was one of the earliest textbooks of dermatologic surgery and covers a broad range of procedures including many cosmetic ones such as hair transplantation. Its design is somewhat traditional but the information is reliable. The photographic quality varies, but for those who would like to round out their skin surgery library, this book is a well-established and readable volume.

Fundamentals of Cutaneous Surgery. Richard G. Bennett. Mosby, St. Louis, MO, 1988.
This substantial book consists of over 800 pages of detailed and erudite surgical information. The graphics are superb and the text is distinguished by its well-written and practical background information. There is much basic science information available to the curious reader as well as superb technical information. This should be considered a standard reference text for the dermatologic surgeon.

Atlas of Cutaneous Surgery, Neil Swanson. Little Brown, Boston, 1988.
This volume is an excellent atlas of dermatologic surgery that permits the reader to develop skills on a step-by-step basis. By using this book in conjunction with the assistance of teaching aids such as pigs' feet, an individual can easily become quite skilled in the rudiments of dermatologic surgery.

Further Reading

Cutaneous Anatomy, Stuart Salasche. Mosby, St. Louis, MO, 1989.
This superb volume details, through excellent graphics, those anatomic structures and relations that are important to the dermatologic surgeon. The text follows the art very closely and details areas of special concern for individuals performing cutaneous surgery.

"Nonexcisional treatment of benign and premalignant cutaneous lesions," G. S. Morganroth and D. J. Leffell. *Clinical Plastic Surgery*, Volume 20, No. 1, January 1993, pages 91–104. The correct diagnosis of benign and premalignant cutaneous lesions requires appropriate biopsy techniques that reflect an understanding of the specific cutaneous pathology. This article discusses biopsy techniques that yield the best functional and cosmetic results.

Color Atlas and Synopsis of Pigmented Lesions. Raymond L. Barnhill. McGraw-Hill Co., New York, 1995.
This small volume is an excellent atlas of pigmented lesions. Its color photographs are very valuable for those who would like to develop diagnostic knowledge. It goes into somewhat greater detail regarding the histopathology than would be required by the general skin surgeon.

Atlas of Cutaneous Surgery, June K. Robinson, K. A. Arndt, P. E. Leboit, and B. U. Wintroub. W. B. Saunders Co., Philadelphia, 1996.
This volume is over 350 pages long and contains very high-quality art and color photographs. Its purpose is to describe in practical detail the elements of cutaneous surgery. The authors represent leaders in the field. In 35 chapters the authors and editors transport us from superficial cutaneous anatomy through electrosurgery and considerations in hemostasis to experimental techniques for repigmentation, graft methods, and other advanced topics. It is an excellent volume and is part of a companion series that represents a comprehensive dermatologic textbook.

Index

A

Absorbable sutures, wound closure materials, 123–126. *See also* Wound closure materials
Accessory nerve, spinal, neck anatomy, 48–49
Acidic preservatives, local anesthesia additives, 85–86
Acquired bleeding diathesis, bleeding complications causes, 184–185
Actinic keratoses, 17–18
Adverse effects, local anesthesia, 87–88
Alcohol, bleeding complications, 185, 188
Allergic reactions:
  local anesthesia, 86
  surgical complications, 199–200
Anatomy, 31–49
  head and neck, 40–49
    blood supply, 47–48
    forehead, 42–47
    generally, 40–42
    neck considerations, 48–49
    sensory nerves, 47, 48
  regional considerations, 34–40
    back and chest, 37, 39
    ears, 35–36
    eyes, 36
    lower extremities, 40
    mouth, 34
    neck, 37
    nose, 34–35
    scalp, 37, 38
    upper extremities, 39–40
  skin
    overview of, 31–32
    relaxed skin tension lines, 32–34
Anesthesia. *See* Local anesthesia
Angioma, 15
Antibiotics:
  contact dermatitis, surgical complications, 198–199
  infection prevention, 194
  prophylaxis, patient preparation, 141–143
Antihistamines, local anesthesia, 86
Antiseptics, excisional surgery, drape and prepping, 154–155
Aspirin, bleeding management, 188
Atrophy, 16
Atypical nevus, 23–25, 206
Autoclaves, surgical instruments, 115

B

Back, anatomy, 37, 39
Basal cell cancer:
  action guide for, 232
  defined, 13, 18–20
  diagnosis and management of, 213
Benign lesions, 26–29
  condyloma, 29

Benign lesions (*Continued*)
  sebaceous hyperplasia, 26
  seborrheic keratoses, 26–27
  skin tags, 27
  solar lentigo, 27–28
  warts, 28–29
Benzocaine, topical anesthesia, 94
Biopsy. *See* Skin biopsy
Black light, 16
Black papule, 15
Bleeding, excisional surgery procedures, 160
Bleeding complications, 181–189
  causes of, 182–185
  generally, 181–182
  management of, 185–187
  prevention of, 187–189
Bleeding diathesis, bleeding complications causes, 184–185
Blister, 15
Blood supply, head anatomy, 47–48
Blood thinners, patient preparation, 143, 147
Blue macule, 9, 11
Blue nevus, 14, 15
Bovine collagen, intraoperative bleeding management, 186
Brown macule, 9, 10
Brown papule, 13, 14

C

Cancers and precancerous lesions, 17–25
  actinic keratoses, 17–18
  basal cell cancer, 18–20, 213
  lentigo maligna, 21, 209–210
  melanoma, 21–23, 205–209
  nevi, 210–212
  squamous cell cancer, 20, 213
Catgut (surgical gut), described, 124
Cautery, bleeding complications causes, 183–184
Cellulitis, 190
Chalazion clamp, described, 113
Cheek, local anesthesia techniques, 93

Chest, anatomy, 37, 39
Chin, local anesthesia techniques, 93
Cigarette smoking, necrosis, surgical complications, 195
Coagulation, wound healing, 52–53
Cocaine, topical anesthesia, 94
Collagen:
  bovine, intraoperative bleeding management, 186
  wound healing, 53–54, 55
Comedone, 13
Complications. *See* Surgical complications
Condyloma, 12, 13, 29
Confidentiality, legal risk management, 228
Contact dermatitis, surgical complications, 198–199
Coumadin (warfarin):
  bleeding complications causes, 182–183
  blood thinners, 143, 147
Crust, 15
Cryoanesthesia, topical anesthesia, 93–94
Cryosurgery, lentigo maligna, 209–210
Curette, described, 111–112
Curette biopsy, described, 68–70
Cysts, 15, 217–219

D

Dacron (polyesters, Mersilene, Ethibond), wound closure materials, 127
Dehiscence, surgical complications, 195–197
Dermatitis, contact, surgical complications, 198–199
Dermatofibroma, 13
Dermatologic disease, incidence of, 3
Dexon (polyglycolic acid), described, 124

Diagnosis:
    benign lesions, 26–29. *See also* Benign lesions
    cancers and precancerous lesions, 17–25. *See also* Cancers and precancerous lesions
    lesion definition, 7–16
    lesion study, 16–17
Diazepam (Valium), preanesthesia medications, 95–96
Dietary restriction, bleeding complications, 185
Digital block, local anesthesia techniques, 91
Diphendydramine, local anesthesia, 86
Documentation:
    legal risk management, 226–227
    skin biopsy, 80–81
Dog ears, wound closure, 172–173, 174–175
Drape and prepping, excisional surgery, 154–156
Dressings:
    bleeding complications, 189
    occlusive, wound healing, 58
    patient preparation, 144–146, 147
    wound closure, 173, 176–177, 178
Drug interactions, local anesthesia, 87–88
Dry field, excisional surgery procedures, 160

E
Ears, anatomy, 35–36
Edema, surgical complications, 202
Electrocautery, bleeding complications causes, 183–184
Electrosurgical equipment, surgical suite, 118
Ellipse, excisional surgery, 152–153, 154
Emergency equipment, surgical suite, 119
Endocarditis prophylaxis, patient preparation, 142

Endogenous bleeding, bleeding complications causes, 184–185
Epidermal cysts, 217–219
Epinephrine:
    intraoperative bleeding management, 186
    local anesthesia additives, 85, 86
    tricyclic antidepressants, drug interactions, 88
Erb's point, neck anatomy, 49
Erosion, 15
Erythema, 16
Ethibond (polyesters, Dacron, Mersilene), wound closure materials, 127
Excisional biopsy:
    incisional biopsy versus, 62–63
    technique for, 74
Excisional surgery, 149–179
    anesthesia, 153–154
    complications. *See* Surgical complications
    drape and prepping, 154–156
    ellipse, 152–153, 154
    lentigo maligna, 209–210
    lesion marking, 151–152
    melanoma, 208–209
    Mohs' surgery, 214–217
    nevi, 210–212
    planning, 149–151
    procedures, 156–161
        generally, 156–158
        hemostasis, 158–159
        infection complications, 192
        tissue handling, 159–160
        undermining, 161
    wound closure, 162–179
        dog ears, 172–173, 174–175
        dressing, 173, 176–177, 178
        generally, 162–171
        Lazy S repair, 171–172
        M-plasty, 172, 173
        specialty sutures, 177
        suture allergy, 179
        suture removal, 177–179
Excisional wound-care instruction, patient preparation, 144

Index

Eye:
  anatomy, 36
  antiseptics, excisional surgery, 155
Eyelid, local anesthesia techniques, 93

F
Face:
  anatomy, 40–48. *See also* Anatomy
  local anesthesia techniques, 93
Facial nerve, head anatomy, 45, 46
Fan distribution, local anesthesia techniques, 89
Fentanyl, preanesthesia medications, 96–97
Fingers:
  local anesthesia techniques, 91–92
  nail biopsy, described, 76–80
Flesh-colored papule, 12, 13
Foot:
  anatomy, 40
  local anesthesia techniques, 90
Forceps, described, 105, 106, 108
Forehead:
  anatomy, 42–47
  local anesthesia techniques, 93

G
Genetic bleeding diathesis, endogenous bleeding, bleeding complications causes, 184–185
Genital condyloma, 12, 13, 29
Giant comedone, 15
Granulating wound-care instruction, patient preparation, 145–146
Granulation, surgical complications, 197–198

H
Halo nervus, 9, 10
Hand, anatomy, 39–40
Healing. *See* Wound healing
Heart, toxic reactions, local anesthesia, 87–88
Hemangioma, 15
Hematoma:
  management of, 187
  prevention of, 184
Hemostasis:
  excisional surgery procedures, 158–159
  incomplete, bleeding complications causes, 183–184
Hemostats, described, 107, 108
Hypergranulation, surgical complications, 197–198
Hypertrophic scar:
  management of, 219, 220
  surgical complications, 200–201
Hypopigmented macule, 9, 10

I
Ice packs, bleeding complications, 185
Incisional biopsy, excisional biopsy versus, 62–63
Indications, patient preparation, 133–134
Infection complications, 189–194
  generally, 189–191
  operative technique, 192
  patient factors, 191
  prevention, 194
  treatment, 193
  wound factors, 192–193
Inflamed seborrheic keratoses, 14
Inflammation phase, wound healing, 52–53
Informed consent:
  legal risk management, 224–226
  patient evaluation, 139, 140, 141
Infraorbital nerve, head anatomy, 48
Infraorbital nerve block, local anesthesia techniques, 93
Instrument stand, surgical suite, 118
Intraoperative bleeding, bleeding management, 185–186

K

Kaposi's sarcoma, 15
Keloids:
  defined, 13
  management of, 219, 220
  surgical complications, 201
Keratoacanthoma, diagnosis and management of, 213–214
Knots, wound closure procedures, 163–164

L

Labial artery, head anatomy, 48
Latex, allergic reaction to, surgical complications, 200
Lazy S repair, wound closure, 171–172
Legal risk management, 223–228
  confidentiality, 228
  documentation, 226–227
  informed consent, 139, 140, 141, 224–226
  overview, 223–224
Lentigo maligna:
  defined, 21, 27
  diagnosis and management, 209–210
Lentigo maligna melanoma, 27
Lesion:
  benign lesions, 26–29. *See also* Benign lesions
  cancers and precancerous lesions, 17–25. *See also* Cancers and precancerous lesions
  definitions, 7–16
  studying of, 16–17
Lesion marking, for excisional surgery, 151–152
Lidocaine:
  allergic reactions, 86
  drug interactions, 88
  local anesthesia, 84, 86
  topical anesthesia, 94
  toxic reactions, 87–88
Lighting, surgical suite, 117–118
Lipomas, management of, 219
Local anesthesia, 83–97
  additives, 85–86
  adverse effects and drug interactions, 87–88
  allergic reactions, 86
  chemistry and classification, 83–84
  excisional surgery procedures, 153–154
  overview, 83
  preanesthesia medications, 95–97
  techniques, 88–93
    digital block, 91
    generally, 88–90
    nerve block, 90–93
    ring block, 90
    trigeminal nerve block, 92, 93
  topical anesthesia, 93–94
  tumescent anesthesia, 94–95
Lower extremities, anatomy, 40

M

Macule, 9–11
Magnifying glass, 16–17
Malignant melanoma. *See* Melanoma
Mandibular nerve, head anatomy, 47
Marking, lesion marking, for excisional surgery, 151–152
Maxon (polytrimethylylene carbonate), described, 125
Medical history, patient preparation, 134–138
Melanin, light and, 16
Melanoma, 205–209
  clinical characteristics, 211
  defined, 13, 21–23
  incidence of, 3, 205
  management of, 208–209
  recognition of, 206, 208
  skin biopsy, 75
  survival data, 207
Melanoma in situ, 27, 206
Mental nerve block, local anesthesia techniques, 93
Meperidine, preanesthesia medications, 96

Index

Mersilene (polyesters, Dacron, Ethibond), wound closure materials, 127
Metastatic tumor, 13
Midazolam (Versed), preanesthesia medications, 96
Mohs' surgery, 214–217
Molluscum contagiosum, 13
Monocryl (poliglecaprone 25), described, 125–126
Mouth, anatomy, 34
M-plasty, wound closure, 172, 173

N

Nail biopsy, described, 76–80
Neck anatomy, 37, 48–49
Necrosis, surgical complications, 194–195
Needle(s):
 materials, 128–130
 procedures, 162
Needle holders, described, 103–104
Nerve block, local anesthesia techniques, 90–93
Nevi:
 described, 12, 13, 14, 23–25, 206
 diagnosis and management, 210–212
Nevus of ota, 11
Nodular basal cell cancer, 19
Nodule, 15
Nonabsorbable sutures, wound closure materials. *See also* Wound closure materials
Nonsteroidal anti-inflammatory drugs, bleeding complications causes, 182
Nose:
 anatomy, 34–35
 local anesthesia techniques, 93
Novafil (Polybutester), wound closure materials, 127
Novocain, allergic reactions, 86
Nylon, wound closure materials, 126–127

O

Occlusive dressings, wound healing, 58
Operative report, documentation, legal risk management, 226–227
Opthalmic nerve, head anatomy, 44
Optical anesthetics, topical anesthesia, 94
Oral biopsy, described, 75–76
Oxygen monitor, surgical suite, 119

P

Pacemakers, patient preparation, 143
Papilloma virus, 28, 29
Papule, 12, 13
Paronychia, 16
Patch, 13
Patient evaluation, described, 138–141
Patient history, infection complications, 191
Patient preparation, 133–147
 bleeding complications, 188–189
 blood thinners, 143, 147
 dressings, 144–146, 147
 indications, 133–134
 medical history, 134–138
 overview, 133
 pacemakers, 143
 patient evaluation, 138–141
 prophylaxis, 141–143
Pharmacology:
 antibiotic prophylaxis, 141–143
 antiseptics, excisional surgery, 154–155
 bleeding complications, 182–183, 186, 188
 contact dermatitis, surgical complications, 198–199
 infection complications
  patient factors, 191
  prevention, 194
  treatment, 193
 local anesthesia, 83–97. *See also* Local anesthesia

preanesthesia medications, 95–97
  wound-healing inhibitory effects, 53
Pigment, scar, surgical complications, 201
Pigmented lesions, action guide for, 231
Plague, 11, 13
Planning, for excisional surgery, 149–151
Plaque, 13
Poliglecaprone 25 (Monocryl), described, 125–126
Polybutester (Novafil), wound closure materials, 127
Polydioxanone (PDS), described, 125
Polyesters (Dacron, Mersilene, Ethibond), wound closure materials, 127
Polyglactin 910 (Vicryl), described, 124–125
Polyglycolic acid (Dexon), described, 124
Polypropylene (Prolene, Surgilene), described, 127
Polysporin, allergic reaction to, surgical complications, 199
Polytrimethylylene carbonate (Maxon), described, 125
Postoperative bleeding, bleeding management, 186–187
Preanesthesia medications, described, 95–97
Prolene (polypropylene, Surgilene), described, 127
Proliferation phase, wound healing, 53–54
Proparacaine, optical anesthesia, 94
Prophylaxis, patient preparation, 141–143
Propranolol, drug interactions, 88
Proud flesh (hypergranulation), surgical complications, 197–198
Pseudomonas infection, 193
Punch, described, 113
Punch biopsy:
  advantages and disadvantages, 62
  described, 70–74
Pustule, 15, 16

R
Record keeping:
  legal risk management, 226–227
  skin biopsy, 80–81
Red macule, 9
Red nodule, 15
Referral, guidelines for, 221
Relaxed skin tension lines, described, 32–34
Rhytids, vertical, mouth anatomy, 34, 35
Ring block, local anesthesia techniques, 90
Risk management. *See* Legal risk management
Rodent ulcer, 19

S
Scab, 15
Scalp:
  anatomy, 37, 38, 43
  suturing of, 161
Scalpel, described, 100–102
Scar:
  legal risk management, 225–226
  management of, 219, 229
  surgical complications, 200–203
  wound closure procedures, 168
  wound healing, 54–57
Scissors, described, 108–111
Scissors biopsy, described, 70, 71
Sebaceous hyperplasia, 26
Seborrheic keratoses:
  defined, 13, 14, 26–27
  inflamed, defined, 14
Second intention healing, wound healing, 57–59
Sensory nerves, head anatomy, 47, 48
Shave biopsy:
  advantages and disadvantages, 62
  described, 63–68

Index

Silk, wound closure materials, 126
Skin:
   cross section of, 8
   overview of, 31–32
   relaxed skin tension lines, 32–34
Skin biopsy, 61–81
   action guide for, 230
   curette biopsy, 68–70
   excisional biopsy technique, 74
   incisional versus excisional biopsy, 62–63
   overview, 61–62
   punch biopsy, 70–74
   record keeping, 80–81
   scissors biopsy, 70, 71
   shave biopsy, 63–68
   special considerations, 75–80
      melanoma, 75
      nail biopsy, 76–80
      oral biopsy, 75–76
Skin hooks:
   described, 105, 107
   excisional surgery procedures, 159
Skin preparation agents, allergic reaction to, surgical complications, 200
Skin surgery. *See* Excisional surgery
Skin tags, 13, 27
Solar lentigo, 9, 27–28
Specialty sutures, wound closure, 177
Spinal accessory nerve, neck anatomy, 48–49
Spread scar, surgical complications, 201
Squamous cell cancer:
   action guide for, 233
   defined, 20
   diagnosis and management of, 213–214
   ears, 36
Staphylococcal infection, 190
Staples, wound closure materials, 131
Sterilization, surgical instruments, 115
Suction, surgical suite, 118
Supraorbital nerve block, local anesthesia techniques, 93
Surgery. *See* Excisional surgery
Surgical complications, 181–203
   action guide for, 234
   bleeding, 181–189
      causes of, 182–185
      generally, 181–182
      management of, 185–187
      prevention of, 187–189
   contact dermatitis, 198–199
   dehiscence, 195–197
   hypergranulation, 197–198
   infection, 189–194
      generally, 189–191
      operative technique, 192
      patient factors, 191
      prevention, 194
      treatment, 193
      wound factors, 192–193
   necrosis, 194–195
   overview, 181, 182
   tape reactions, 199
Surgical gut (catgut), described, 124
Surgical instruments, 99–119
   care of, 113–115
   chalazion clamp, 113
   curette, 111–112
   forceps, 105, 106, 108
   hemostats, 107, 108
   needle holders, 103–104
   overview, 99–100
   punch, 113
   scalpels, 100–102
   scissors, 108–111
   skin hooks, 105, 107
   towel clip, 113
   vendors listed, 235–237
Surgical knots, wound closure procedures, 163–164
Surgical preparation. *See* Patient preparation
Surgical suite, 115–119
   chair, 117
   electrosurgical equipment, 118
   emergency equipment, 119

instrument stand, 118
lighting, 117–118
oxygen monitor, 119
requirements, 115–116
suction, 118
table, 116–117
vendors listed, 235–237
waste disposal, 118
Surgical wound healing. *See*
  Wound healing
Surgilene (polypropylene, Prolene),
  described, 127
Suture and suturing:
  allergy, wound closure, 179
  materials. *See* Wound closure
    materials
  removal, wound closure,
    177–179
  of scalp, 161
  surgical complications, 202–203
  wound closure, 162–179. *See also*
    Wound closure

T
Talon noir, 9, 10
Tape reactions, surgical
  complications, 199
Telangiectasis, scar, surgical
  complications, 201
Temporal artery, head anatomy,
  43
Temporal nerve, head anatomy, 45,
  46
Tetracaine, optical anesthesia, 94
Thick scar, surgical complications,
  200–201
Thrombin, intraoperative bleeding
  management, 186
Tissue handling, excisional surgery
  procedures, 159–160
Toes, nail biopsy, described, 76–80
Topical anesthesia, described,
  93–94
Towel clip, described, 113
Toxic reactions, local anesthesia,
  87–88
Tricyclic antidepressants, drug
  interactions, 88

Trigeminal nerve block, local
  anesthesia techniques, 92, 93
Tumescent anesthesia, described,
  94–95

U
Ulcer, 15
Ultrasonic cleaning, surgical
  instruments, 115
Undermining, excisional surgery
  procedures, 161
Upper extremities, anatomy, 39–40

V
Valium (diazepam), preanesthesia
  medications, 95–96
Vasoconstrictors, local anesthesia
  additives, 85
Vasovagal reactions, toxic
  reactions, 88
Versed (midazolam), preanesthesia
  medications, 96
Vertical rhytids, mouth anatomy,
  34, 35
Vesicle, 15
Vicryl (polyglactin 910), described,
  124–125
Vitiligo, 9, 10

W
Warfarin (Coumadin):
  bleeding complications causes,
    182–183
  blood thinners, 143, 147
Warts, 28–29
Waste disposal, surgical suite, 118
Wedge biopsy, described, 63
Wood's light, 16
Wound-care instruction:
  bleeding complications, 188–189
  patient preparation, 144–146
Wound closure, 162–179
  dressings, 173, 176–177, 178
  generally, 162–171
  suture allergy, 179
  suture removal, 177–179
Wound closure materials, 121–131
  absorbable sutures, 123–126

Wound closure materials (*Continued*)
  catgut (surgical gut), 124
  generally, 123–124
  poliglecaprone 25 (Monocryl), 125–126
  polydioxanone (PDS), 125
  polyglactin 910 (Vicryl), 124–125
  polyglycolic acid (Dexon), 124
  polytrimethylylene carbonate (Maxon), 125
 needles, 128–130
 nonabsorbable sutures, 126–127
  generally, 126
  nylon, 126–127
  polybutester (Novafil), 127
  polyesters (Dacron, Mersilene, Ethibond), 127
  polypropylene (Prolene, Surgilene), 127
  silk, 126
 overview and characteristics of, 121–123
 staples, 131
Wound healing, 51–59
 inflammation phase, 52–53
 overview, 51–52
 pharmacology, inhibitory effects, 53
 proliferation phase, 53–54
 scar, 54–57
 second intention healing, 57–59
Wound separation (dehiscence), surgical complications, 195–197